The Nutritional Healer

Creating Wellness with Better Food Choices

By

ALICE DEE

First Edition

Copyright © 2023 Alice Dee

www.NutritionalHealer.com

www.PeakPerformanceDiet.com

www.TheFoodForestGuide.com

www.RawFromTheGarden.com

Raw From the Garden Press

ISBN: 9798863232508

DEDICATION

This book is gratefully dedicated to the love of my life.

ACKNOWLEDGEMENTS

I wish to acknowledge my many teachers who shared the invaluable information contained in this book with me and encouraged me to write about it so that others can benefit from and heal their lives using it.

TABLE OF CONTENTS

PREFACE

As you embark on a path to better health accompanied by "The Nutritional Healer: Creating Wellness with Better Food Choices," I am thrilled to share with you the wisdom and insights that have transformed my own life and the lives of countless others. This book is a labor of love—a culmination of years of exploration, study, and personal experience that has led me to a profound understanding of the healing power of nutrition, particularly the remarkable health benefits of a raw plant-based diet.

Although my higher educational studies were centered on the physical sciences, my research into the world of nutritional healing began not as a pursuit of a career but as a quest for personal well-being. Like many, I faced health challenges and excess weight that left me searching for answers beyond conventional medicine. I was fortunate to stumble upon the idea that food could be more than just sustenance; it could be medicine—a source of vitality, healing, and physical transformation.

In my early days of discovery, I encountered the science-based notion that humans are, at their core, physiological frugivores. This perspective resonated deeply with me and led me to explore the profound connection between our evolutionary heritage and our dietary choices. It was a revelation to realize that the foods that have sustained our species for millennia could hold the keys to unlocking radiant health and well-being.

The idea of consuming an entirely plant-based diet, abundant in fresh raw foods, captivated my imagination and became the foundation of my personal wellness journey. As I delved deeper into this dietary path, I witnessed remarkable changes in my own health—increased energy, improved digestion, welcome weight loss, remarkable happiness, mental clarity, and a sense of vitality that I had never before experienced. I knew I was onto something extraordinary!

This remarkable experience gave me all the encouragement I needed to open a pioneering raw vegan restaurant to share my healing experience with others since it wasn't enough for me to keep this knowledge to myself. I felt compelled to share what I had learned with others who, like me, were seeking a path to wellness that aligned with their own bodies and the natural world.

With that background and decades of subsequent study into the healing value of the most natural diet for humans, "The Nutritional Healer" was born—a book written to serve as a guide, a companion, and a source of inspiration for those who wish to embark on their own path toward nutritional healing.

The Wisdom of a Raw Plant-Based Diet

At the heart of this book lies the profound concept of using a raw plant-based diet as a means of nourishing our bodies and unlocking their inherent potential for healing. You will be introduced to the compelling concept that our evolutionary history as physiological frugivores provides us with a science-based blueprint for dietary choices that resonate with our biology and our deepest well-being.

Raw plant foods, with their vibrant colors, rich flavors, and life-giving nutrients, take center stage in this dietary approach. Learn to celebrate the variety of flavors and textures that fresh fruits, vegetables, nuts, and seeds can bring to your plate. Delve into the science of enzymes and their role in supporting digestion and overall vitality, and revel in the beauty of foods that are both healing and delicious.

The healing potential of a high raw plant-based diet is not a mere promise but a reality grounded in both ancient wisdom and modern science. Explore the scientific evidence that highlights the protective effects of plant-based foods against chronic diseases, the anti-inflammatory properties of phytonutrients, and the positive impact a diet rich in them has on heart health, weight management, and mental well-being.

As you study the chapters of this book, you will find practical guidance on how to embrace this dietary path in a way that suits your individual preferences and lifestyle. You'll discover tips for mindful eating, strategies for grocery shopping and meal planning, and the joy of preparing nourishing, plant-based meals. You'll also gain insight into the importance of creating a supportive food environment that nurtures your wellness goals.

The Intelligent Use of Supplements

While a raw plant-based diet forms the cornerstone of our approach to nutritional healing since it is generally far more abundant in ephemeral micronutrients than other diets, this dietary program also recognizes the need for flexibility and adaptation. There may thus be instances where intelligent and justified supplementation is necessary to correct any nutritional deficiencies that can arise over time.

This book explores the science behind micronutrient supplements and their role in supporting optimal health and healing. Explore the nuanced considerations that go into supplementing your diet given the understanding that it should always be done with wisdom and intention.

When it comes to using supplements, the overall aim of this book is to provide you with the knowledge to make informed decisions about them, ensuring that they complement your dietary choices and supports your overall wellness.

A Path to Wellness

Keep in mind that "The Nutritional Healer" is more than just a book; it is a roadmap that leads you to the heart of your well-being, the essence of your vitality, the wisdom of your body, and your place in nature. It offers a path of self-discovery, empowerment, and transformation should you choose to take it. It can bring you from where you are today to a place of greater health, joy, and vibrancy.

As you turn the pages of this book, I encourage you to approach your exploration of nutritional healing with an open heart and a curious mind. The path may be unfamiliar at times, but know that you are not alone. I am here as your guide, your companion, and your fellow traveler on this transformative healing adventure.

I now invite you to embrace the power of nutritional healing, to celebrate the life-giving potential of a raw plant-based diet, and to make informed choices that support your health and the well-being of our planet and fellow creatures. Together, we can create a brighter, more vibrant future—one where wellness is not just a destination but a way of life. To your health!

Alice Dee

INTRODUCTION

NOURISHING YOUR BODY, HEALING YOUR LIFE

In an age where wellness is not merely a trend but a pursuit of profound significance, the healing potential of our daily choices is undeniable. This book will take you on a fascinating journey that will illuminate the extraordinary power for creating or destroying health that resides within the foods we choose to consume.

This book is an invitation to explore a nutritional path that resonates with our evolutionary heritage and modern scientific understanding—a path that harnesses the vitality of a plant-based diet that contains a generous infusion of fresh raw foods.

In the labyrinth of dietary theories and nutritional philosophies that populate our world today, we pause to explore a perspective rooted in our physiological and psychological design.

We delve into the notion that, at our core, humans are, to a significant degree, physiological frugivores—creatures biologically primed to thrive on a diet predominantly composed of plant foods, especially fruits.

The essence of this nutritional journey is the embrace of an entirely plant-based diet, a dietary choice that has been celebrated for its profound healing potential. In the following pages, we will explore how this lifestyle choice can not only promote physical health but also nurture emotional well-being and environmental harmony.

By adopting a diet rich in colorful fruits, leafy greens, vegetables, grains, nuts, and seeds as nature provides them in their raw state, we embark on a path that aligns with the natural needs of our bodies and the innate wisdom of our ancestors' dietary patterns.

But our exploration doesn't end there. We also acknowledge that in our complex world, achieving optimal nutrition can sometimes require intelligent and justified supplementation.

We recognize that deficiencies can manifest over time, leading to various forms of unwellness. With the guidance of scientific knowledge, we will explore the responsible use of supplements to address these imbalances, ensuring that we maintain a state of vibrant health throughout our lives.

As we journey through the pages of this book, you will discover the profound impact that our food choices have on our physical, mental, and emotional well-being.

You will learn about the nutrients that sustain us, the foods that heal us, and the dietary practices that promote longevity and vitality. We will explore the art of mindful eating, the joy of preparing wholesome meals, and the profound connection between what we eat and how we feel.

"The Nutritional Healer" is a testament to the transformative power of conscious, deliberate choices—choices that can pave the way for a life brimming with health and vitality.

So, let us embark on this journey together, unraveling the secrets of nutritional healing, and forging a path toward a future where we are not just consumers of food but stewards of our own well-being, the well-being of the planet and the well-being of our fellow creatures.

It's time to nourish your body, heal your life, and create a brighter, more vibrant tomorrow!

THE POWER OF NUTRITION IN HEALING

In the grand tapestry of life, the role of nutrition is a thread that weaves its way through every aspect of our existence. It is a force that influences not only the course of our physical health but also the quality of our emotional and mental well-being.

Nutrition is not merely about satisfying our hunger or pleasing our palate; it is the cornerstone of our vitality, the foundation upon which our very lives are built. In this section, we embark on a journey to explore the profound and transformative power of nutrition in healing, with a particular focus on the benefits of a high raw plant-based diet.

The Healing Potential of Food

The notion that food can be a powerful agent of healing is not a recent revelation. Ancient civilizations across the globe have long recognized the therapeutic properties of various foods and herbs.

From the Ayurvedic tradition in India to Traditional Chinese Medicine, and even among Native American cultures, there is a shared belief that food is medicine. In these traditions, diet was seen not just as a means of sustenance but as a pathway to health and wellness.

In our modern world, we have witnessed a resurgence of interest in the healing potential of food. Scientific research has brought to light the intricate ways in which the nutrients found in our diet interact with our bodies, influencing our health at the cellular level.

The recognition of the link between diet and disease has led to a paradigm shift in how we perceive nutrition. Food is no longer seen as mere calories to fuel our activities but as a dynamic force capable of preventing, mitigating, and even reversing chronic illnesses.

A fundamental concept in the healing power of food is the idea of "food as information." Every morsel we eat sends a message to our genes, cells, and organs. The quality of that information can either promote health or contribute to disease.

When we consume whole, plant-based foods, especially in their raw and unprocessed state, we are providing our bodies with a symphony of nutrients and phytonutrients—natural compounds found in plants that have a myriad of health-promoting effects.

The Raw Advantage: A Return to Our Roots

In our quest to harness the healing potential of nutrition, we find ourselves drawn back to our evolutionary roots. As physiological frugivores, our ancestors predominantly consumed fruits and plants as their primary source of sustenance. This dietary choice was not merely a matter of availability but a reflection of our biological design. The human body is uniquely adapted to thrive on the nourishing abundance of the plant kingdom.

One of the key principles that underlie the healing potential of a high raw plant-based diet is the preservation of the vital nutrients found in foods. Heat, especially at high temperatures, can destroy or alter many of these essential compounds. Raw foods, on the other hand, retain their natural integrity, offering a potent concentration of vitamins, minerals, enzymes, and phytonutrients that are essential for our health.

When we consume raw plant foods, we are not only providing our bodies with a rich source of nutrients but also aiding our digestive system. Raw foods are teeming with digestive enzymes that assist in breaking down the foods we eat, making the absorption of nutrients more efficient. This natural synergy between our bodies and raw plant foods is a testament to the alignment between our biology and the foods that have sustained us for millennia.

A Symphony of Colors and Flavors

A high raw plant-based diet is a celebration of diversity—a vibrant tapestry of colors, textures, and flavors that invigorate our senses and nourish our bodies. It is a diet that encourages us to savor the natural sweetness of ripe fruits, the crispness of fresh vegetables, and the richness of nuts and seeds.

It is a diet that invites us to explore the boundless variety of nature's offerings, from the delicate petals of edible flowers to the robustness of leafy greens.

Each color in the plant kingdom corresponds to a unique set of phytonutrients, each with its own healing properties. For instance, the deep orange of carrots and sweet potatoes signifies the presence of beta-carotene, a potent antioxidant that supports eye health and boosts our immune system. The vibrant red of tomatoes and strawberries heralds the presence of lycopene, known for its potential in reducing the risk of certain cancers.

The flavors found in raw plant foods are a testament to the richness of our natural world. From the tartness of citrus fruits to the creaminess of avocados, each taste offers a unique culinary experience while providing our bodies with essential nutrients. Raw foods are alive with flavor, and when we embrace them, we embark on a journey of culinary exploration that is as satisfying as it is nourishing.

Food Synergy: The Magic of Whole Foods

In our pursuit of health, it's not just the individual nutrients in our food that matter but also how they interact with each other. Whole, unprocessed foods offer a symphony of nutrients that work in harmony to promote optimal health. This phenomenon is known as food synergy.

Consider, for example, the humble tomato. While lycopene, a powerful antioxidant, is often credited for its health benefits, consuming a whole tomato provides a broader spectrum of nutrients, including vitamins C and K, potassium, and folate. These nutrients complement each other, enhancing the overall health-promoting effects of the tomato.

The same principle applies to a high raw plant-based diet. When we consume a variety of raw fruits, vegetables, nuts, and seeds, we are not just obtaining individual nutrients; we are creating a symphony of healing compounds that support our well-being in multifaceted ways. It's as if nature, in its wisdom, has designed these foods to nourish us comprehensively.

Unlocking the Potential of Enzymes

Enzymes are the unsung heroes of our digestive system. They are responsible for breaking down the foods we eat into smaller, absorbable molecules that our bodies can use for energy and repair. The presence of enzymes in raw plant foods is a key factor in their healing potential.

When we cook food at high temperatures, we often destroy these vital enzymes, making digestion more taxing on our bodies. Raw foods, in contrast, are brimming with enzymes that support our digestive processes. This natural aid to digestion can alleviate common issues such as bloating, gas, and indigestion, allowing us to enjoy our meals without discomfort.

In addition to aiding digestion, enzymes play a role in reducing inflammation and supporting detoxification. For instance, the enzyme bromelain, found in pineapples, has been studied for its potential to reduce inflammation and promote tissue healing. Another enzyme, papain, derived from papayas, has been used for its digestive and anti-inflammatory properties.

A High Raw Plant-Based Diet and Inflammation

Chronic inflammation is now recognized as a key driver of many chronic diseases, including heart disease, diabetes, and cancer. It's a silent fire within our bodies that, when left unchecked, can lead to tissue damage and long-term health problems. But our dietary choices can either fuel this inflammation or extinguish its flames.

A high raw plant-based diet is a natural anti-inflammatory diet. Raw fruits and vegetables are rich in antioxidants, which combat the oxidative stress that fuels inflammation. They are also abundant in phytonutrients that have been shown to have anti-inflammatory properties. For instance, curcumin, found in turmeric, has potent anti-inflammatory effects and has been studied extensively for its potential in reducing inflammation.

The fiber in raw plant foods also plays a role in reducing inflammation. It nourishes our gut microbiota, the community of microorganisms living in our digestive tract, which in turn influences our immune system and inflammation levels. A healthy gut microbiota, fostered by a diet rich in fiber, can help regulate inflammation and support overall health.

A Nourished Mind: The Connection Between Diet and Mental Health

While the physical benefits of a high raw plant-based diet are well-documented, the impact on mental health is equally profound. Our brains, like the rest of our bodies, depend on the nutrients we consume to function optimally. The foods we eat can either support mental clarity, emotional well-being, and cognitive function, or they can contribute to brain fog, mood swings, and even mental health disorders.

Research has shown that certain nutrients found abundantly in raw plant foods are particularly beneficial for the brain. Omega-3 fatty acids, for example, found in flaxseeds, walnuts, and chia seeds, are essential for brain health and have been linked to improved mood and cognitive function.

Furthermore, antioxidants in fruits and vegetables protect the brain from oxidative stress, which has been implicated in conditions such as depression and Alzheimer's disease.

Moreover, the gut-brain connection is gaining recognition as a crucial link between diet and mental health. The gut microbiota, influenced by the foods we eat, communicates with the brain through a complex network known as the gut-brain axis.

The composition of our gut microbiota can influence our mood, stress response, and even our risk of mental health disorders. A diet rich in raw plant foods that nourishes a diverse and healthy gut microbiota can contribute to a positive mental outlook.

The Healing Power of Plant-Based Proteins

One common concern when transitioning to a high raw plant-based diet is protein intake. However, this concern is often misplaced. Plant-based foods offer a wealth of protein sources that are not only abundant but also incredibly healthful.

Legumes such as lentils, chickpeas, and black beans are excellent sources of plant-based protein. They are not only rich in protein but also provide essential nutrients like fiber, vitamins, and minerals. Nuts and seeds, including almonds, hemp seeds, pumpkin seeds, and chia seeds, are also protein powerhouses. Incorporating these foods into a high raw plant-based diet ensures that you meet your protein needs without the saturated fat and cholesterol often associated with animal-based sources.

In addition to protein quantity, it's important to consider protein quality. Plant-based proteins come with a bonus—the absence of harmful saturated fats and cholesterol found in animal products. This means that when you choose plant-based proteins, you are not only meeting your protein requirements but also supporting heart health and reducing your risk of chronic diseases.

Moreover, the amino acids found in plant-based proteins, when combined thoughtfully in a varied diet, provide all the essential amino acids needed for optimal health. The idea of "protein combining" has been debunked, as our bodies are remarkably efficient at utilizing the amino acids from different plant sources to meet our protein needs.

A High Raw Plant-Based Diet: A Path to Weight Wellness

Weight management is a concern for many in today's world, and a high raw plant-based diet can be a powerful ally in achieving and maintaining a healthy weight. One of the key reasons for this lies in the natural balance of nutrients found in raw plant foods.

First and foremost, raw plant foods are generally lower in calories than processed and animal-based foods. This means you can enjoy larger portions of nutrient-dense foods without excessive calorie intake. The fiber in raw plant foods also plays a role in promoting satiety, helping you feel full and satisfied with your meals.

Moreover, raw plant foods are rich in complex carbohydrates, which provide a steady source of energy without the rapid spikes and crashes associated with refined sugars. These carbohydrates, found in fruits, vegetables, and whole grains, fuel your activities and workouts, supporting an active lifestyle that is essential for weight wellness.

The natural combination of fiber, water, and nutrients in raw plant foods also supports healthy digestion, which is crucial for efficient calorie absorption and the elimination of waste. This promotes regularity and reduces the likelihood of constipation, a common issue that can contribute to discomfort and weight gain.

Furthermore, the antioxidants and phytonutrients in raw plant foods play a role in reducing inflammation, which has been linked to weight gain and difficulty losing weight. A diet rich in these compounds can help address underlying factors that contribute to weight-related health issues.

Sustainable Eating for a Thriving Planet

As we delve deeper into the healing potential of a high raw plant-based diet, we cannot ignore the profound impact our dietary choices have on the planet we call home. The global food system is at a critical juncture, with the need for sustainable and environmentally conscious choices becoming increasingly urgent.

Animal agriculture, with its enormous land and resource requirements, is a leading contributor to deforestation, greenhouse gas emissions, and habitat destruction. By choosing a plant-based diet, especially one that emphasizes raw foods, we reduce our ecological footprint and play a part in preserving our natural world for future generations.

Raw plant-based foods have another unique advantage in terms of sustainability: they often require less energy and resources to produce and transport compared to heavily processed foods or animal products. This means that a high raw plant-based diet aligns not only with our health and well-being but also with the health of our planet.

The Science of Nutritional Healing

While the principles of a high raw plant-based diet are rooted in our biological heritage and the wisdom of traditional cultures, modern science continues to provide us with a deeper understanding of how nutrition influences our health.

Throughout this book you can find science-based references at the end of each chapter. These are intended to help satisfy your curiosity and any desire you may have to see the firm scientific foundation upon which the sound nutritional principles presented in the preceding chapter were based.

Furthermore, research in fields such as nutrigenomics—the study of how our genes interact with nutrients—reveals the intricate ways in which our dietary choices can impact our genetic expression and, consequently, our health outcomes.

The field of nutritional epidemiology, which investigates the relationships between diet and disease on a population scale, has provided us with valuable insights into the associations between diet and conditions such as heart disease, cancer, and diabetes.

The evidence consistently points to the protective effects of diets rich in plant-based foods, especially when consumed in their raw and unprocessed form.

Furthermore, advances in the study of the gut microbiota and its role in health have shed light on the importance of our dietary choices in shaping our internal ecosystem.

A high raw plant-based diet, with its emphasis on fiber-rich foods, nourishes a diverse and healthy gut microbiota, which in turn supports our immune system, regulates inflammation, and influences our risk of chronic diseases.

The Art of Nutritional Healing

In this exploration of the power of nutrition in healing, we have journeyed from the origins of our dietary heritage to the frontiers of modern nutritional science. We have uncovered the healing potential of raw plant-based foods, celebrated the synergy of nutrients found in whole foods, and marveled at the profound impact of our dietary choices on our bodies and the planet.

As we continue our voyage through the pages of this book, we will delve even deeper into the practical aspects of embracing a high raw plant-based diet. We will explore the art of mindful eating, the joy of preparing wholesome meals, and the profound connection between what we eat and how we feel. We will also discuss the intelligent and justified use of supplements to correct any deficiencies that may arise over time.

Still, most importantly, we will embark on a journey of self-discovery—a journey that leads to a state of wellness that extends far beyond the physical realm.

Basically, the power of nutrition in healing is not merely a matter of science; it is a testament to the healing power of nature. It also demonstrates that when humans consume the most natural foods for their physiology in the raw state that nature provides them to us, it tends to lead us on the path to our best physical, mental, and spiritual health.

PART I: UNDERSTANDING NUTRITION

UNVEILING THE SCIENCE OF NUTRITIONAL HEALING

In this section on understanding nutrition, we embark on a fascinating journey into the world of food and its value to our bodies and health—an exploration that forms the foundation of our quest for healing through a raw plant-based diet.

We will delve deep into the science of nutrition, unraveling the intricacies of how our bodies interact with the foods we consume and why a plant-based diet, rich in raw foods, is uniquely suited to support our health and well-being.

The Basics of Nutrition

To understand the profound healing potential of a high raw plant-based diet, we must first grasp the fundamentals of nutrition. This knowledge is not only empowering but also serves as the compass that guides our dietary choices. In this section, we'll embark on a comprehensive exploration of the basics of nutrition, laying the groundwork for our journey to wellness.

Nutrition: More Than Just Calories

Nutrition is the science of how our bodies obtain and utilize the substances necessary for life. It's the study of the nutrients in the foods we eat and how these nutrients impact our health. Nutrition goes beyond mere sustenance; it is the cornerstone of our vitality, the source of our energy, and the key to our well-being.

At its core, nutrition is about providing our bodies with the essential elements they need to function optimally. These elements, known as nutrients, can be broadly categorized into two main types: macronutrients and micronutrients.

Macronutrients: Fuel for Your Body

Macronutrients are the nutrients we need in larger quantities to provide our bodies with energy and support growth, repair, and daily functioning. There are three primary macronutrients: carbohydrates, proteins, and fats.

Carbohydrates: The Energy Source

Carbohydrates are the body's preferred source of energy. They are broken down into glucose, a simple sugar, which fuels our cells and provides the energy needed for physical activity and metabolic processes. Carbohydrates are found in a wide variety of foods, including grains, fruits, vegetables, legumes, and even some nuts and seeds.

In a high raw plant-based diet, carbohydrates are primarily derived from fruits and vegetables. These natural sources of carbohydrates are rich in fiber, vitamins, minerals, and antioxidants. They provide sustained energy and promote satiety, making them an ideal choice for those seeking vitality and well-being.

The idea that carbohydrates are an essential part of our diet aligns with the concept that humans are physiological frugivores. Throughout our evolutionary history, fruits, with their natural sweetness and energy-rich content, have been a staple in our diet. Choosing whole, raw fruits as a primary source of carbohydrates supports not only our energy needs but also our overall health.

Proteins: Building Blocks of Life

Proteins are fundamental to life itself. They are the building blocks of tissues, muscles, enzymes, hormones, and virtually every structure in our bodies. Proteins are composed of amino acids, which are essential for growth, repair, and the synthesis of important molecules.

While it is true that animal products are rich sources of protein, they also typically contain an excessive amount of saturated fat and cholesterol that are unnatural and unhealthy for humans to consume since they cause vascular disease that then leads to a host of chronic and even deadly health issues.

It's also essential to recognize that plant-based foods also provide ample protein. In fact, all essential amino acids—the amino acids our bodies cannot produce on their own—are readily available in plant-based sources.

In a high raw plant-based diet, proteins are sourced from a variety of foods, including legumes (such as lentils, chickpeas, and beans), nuts, seeds, and even leafy greens. These plant-based proteins offer numerous advantages— they are typically lower in saturated fat and cholesterol, and they come bundled with an array of phytonutrients, fiber, and antioxidants that support our health.

Fats: Essential for Health

Although fats are often vilified in popular discourse and humans have to be unusually careful to select the right type and amount of fats to consume, fats remain essential for our health. They play crucial roles in the structure of our cell membranes, the absorption of fat-soluble vitamins (such as A, D, E, and K), and the regulation of various bodily functions. Fats are also a concentrated source of energy.

In a high raw plant-based diet, fats are primarily sourced from plant-based foods like avocados, nuts, seeds, and olives. These fats are predominantly unsaturated and rich in monounsaturated and polyunsaturated fatty acids, which have been linked to heart health and the reduction of LDL (low-density lipoprotein) cholesterol—the "bad" cholesterol.

The omega-3 fatty acids, specifically alpha-linolenic acid (ALA), found in flaxseeds, chia seeds, and walnuts, are particularly important for brain health and reducing inflammation.

These fats are an integral part of a balanced diet and can be readily obtained from plant-based sources. Furthermore, those who cannot readily convert ALA to the EPA and DHA needed for brain health and memory can easily supplement with algal oil made from marine algae.

Micronutrients: Vitamins and Minerals

Micronutrients are the essential vitamins and minerals our bodies need in smaller quantities to perform a wide range of biochemical processes. They act as cofactors in enzymatic reactions, antioxidants that combat oxidative stress, and regulators of various physiological functions.

A high raw plant-based diet is rich in micronutrients, providing an abundance of vitamins and minerals that support our health. Let's explore some of the key micronutrients found in plant-based foods:

Vitamins

- **Vitamin C**: Abundant in fruits like oranges, strawberries, and kiwis, vitamin C is essential for immune function, skin health, and wound healing. It also acts as an antioxidant, protecting our cells from damage.
- **Vitamin A**: Found in carrots, sweet potatoes, and dark leafy greens, vitamin A is crucial for vision, immune function, and skin health. It is a fat-soluble vitamin, so consuming these foods with a source of healthy fats enhances its absorption.
- **Vitamin K**: Leafy greens like kale, spinach, and Swiss chard are excellent sources of vitamin K, which is essential for blood clotting and bone health.
- **B Vitamins**: Plant-based foods provide a wide range of B vitamins, including folate (B9), found in leafy greens and legumes; vitamin B6, found in bananas and potatoes; and vitamin B12, which can be obtained through fortified plant-based foods or supplements.

Minerals

- **Calcium**: While dairy products are often associated with calcium, plant-based sources like collard greens, bok choy, almonds, and fortified plant-based milk provide this essential mineral. Calcium is crucial for bone health, muscle function, and nerve transmission.
- **Iron**: Plant-based sources of iron include lentils, chickpeas, tofu, and spinach. Iron from plant foods is non-heme iron, which is less readily absorbed than heme iron from animal products. However, consuming vitamin C-rich foods alongside iron-rich foods enhances iron absorption.
- **Magnesium**: Nuts, seeds, whole grains, and leafy greens are excellent sources of magnesium, which is involved in hundreds of biochemical reactions in the body, including energy production and muscle function.
- **Zinc**: Legumes, nuts, seeds, and whole grains provide zinc, which is essential for immune function, wound healing, and DNA

synthesis.

Phytonutrients: The Healing Compounds in Plants

Beyond macronutrients and micronutrients, plants offer a treasure trove of phytonutrients—natural compounds with remarkable healing properties. Phytonutrients are responsible for the vibrant colors, flavors, and aromas of plant-based foods, and they play a significant role in promoting our health. They include:

- **Carotenoids**: Carotenoids are pigments found in orange, red, and yellow fruits and vegetables, as well as some dark leafy greens. They include beta-carotene, lycopene, and zeaxanthin, among others. Carotenoids act as antioxidants, protecting our cells from oxidative stress, and some can be converted into vitamin A, supporting our vision and immune function.
- **Flavonoids**: Flavonoids are a diverse group of phytonutrients found in foods like citrus fruits, berries, onions, and tea. They have antioxidant and anti-inflammatory properties, contributing to heart health and potentially reducing the risk of chronic diseases.
- **Glucosinolates**: Glucosinolates are sulfur-containing compounds found in cruciferous vegetables like broccoli, kale, and cauliflower. They have been studied for their potential in reducing the risk of certain cancers and supporting liver detoxification.
- **Phytoestrogens**: Phytoestrogens are plant compounds found in foods like soybeans, flaxseeds, and whole grains. They can mimic the hormone estrogen in the body and have been studied for their potential in reducing menopausal symptoms and supporting bone health.
- **Polyphenols**: Polyphenols are abundant in foods like berries, cocoa, and green tea. They have antioxidant and anti-inflammatory properties, contributing to heart health and potentially reducing the risk of chronic diseases.
- **Resveratrol**: Resveratrol is found in grapes and certain berries. It has garnered attention for its potential in supporting heart health and longevity.

Understanding the Healing Potential of Phytonutrients

The healing potential of phytonutrients is a testament to the power of whole, plant-based foods. These compounds not only protect our cells from damage but also interact with our biology in profound ways, influencing gene expression, cellular communication, and various metabolic processes.

In a high raw plant-based diet, we are blessed with an abundance of phytonutrients. Raw fruits and vegetables, in particular, are teeming with these healing compounds, as they are most concentrated in the natural, unprocessed state of the foods.

When we consume raw plant foods, we are not only nourishing our bodies with essential nutrients but also infusing them with the therapeutic properties of phytonutrients.

Enjoying a Variety of Colors and Flavors

One of the remarkable aspects of a high raw plant-based diet is the diversity of colors and flavors that grace our plates. Each color in the plant kingdom corresponds to a unique set of phytonutrients, each with its own healing properties. Here are some examples:

- **Red and Pink:** These colors often signify the presence of anthocyanins, which have antioxidant and anti-inflammatory properties. Foods like strawberries, raspberries, and watermelon boast these vibrant hues.
- **Orange and Yellow:** The pigments in orange and yellow fruits and vegetables, such as carrots and bell peppers, are due to carotenoids like beta-carotene. These compounds support eye health, immune function, and skin health.
- **Green:** Chlorophyll, the pigment responsible for the green color of leafy greens and other vegetables, has been studied for its potential in detoxification and cancer prevention.
- **Purple and Blue:** Blueberries and grapes, with their deep blue and purple hues, contain anthocyanins and resveratrol, which are associated with heart health and longevity.
- **White and Brown:** Garlic and onions, with their characteristic pungency, contain sulfur compounds like allicin, known for their potential in reducing the risk of heart disease and supporting immune function.

When we consume a wide variety of colorful, raw plant foods, we are creating a symphony of healing compounds that work in harmony to promote our well-being. This dietary approach is a celebration of nature's abundance and a testament to the intelligence of whole foods.

Food Synergy: The Magic of Whole Foods

The healing potential of plant-based nutrition is not just about individual nutrients but also how these nutrients interact with each other when consumed as part of whole foods. This phenomenon is known as food synergy.

Food synergy recognizes that the combination of nutrients in whole foods often has a greater impact on our health than individual nutrients in isolation. When we eat whole, unprocessed foods, we are benefiting from the harmonious interplay of vitamins, minerals, fiber, and phytonutrients. Here are some examples of food synergy:

- **Tomatoes**: While lycopene, a powerful antioxidant, is often credited for its health benefits, consuming a whole tomato provides a broader spectrum of nutrients, including vitamins C and K, potassium, and folate. These nutrients complement each other, enhancing the overall health-promoting effects of the tomato.
- **Leafy Greens and Citrus Fruits**: The vitamin C in citrus fruits enhances the absorption of iron from leafy greens. This combination is a prime example of how the right pairing of foods can optimize nutrient utilization in the body.
- **Whole Grains and Legumes**: Combining whole grains and legumes provides a complementary set of amino acids, creating a complete protein source. This is a key principle in plant-based diets, ensuring that we obtain all the essential amino acids we need for health.
- **Nuts and Seeds with Leafy Greens**: The healthy fats in nuts and seeds enhance the absorption of fat-soluble vitamins like A, D, E, and K found in leafy greens. This pairing ensures that we maximize the benefits of these vitamins in our diet.

The Art of Nutritional Healing

As we dive deeper into the world of nutrition, we not only gain knowledge but also cultivate a deep appreciation for the wisdom of our bodies and the natural world. We begin to see food not just as a means of sustenance but as a conduit for healing, a source of vitality, and a pathway to wellness.

In the chapters that follow, we will continue to unravel the mysteries of nutrition, exploring the profound connection between what we eat and how we feel. We will delve into the intelligent and justified use of supplements to correct any deficiencies that may arise over time. And, most importantly, we will embark on a journey of self-discovery—a journey that leads to a state of wellness that extends far beyond the physical realm.

As we navigate the terrain of nutritional healing, remember that you hold the power to make choices that support your health and well-being. The knowledge you gain here is a tool—a tool that empowers you to take charge of your health and embark on a transformative journey toward a brighter, more vibrant future.

With each bite of fresh, raw plant-based food, you nourish your body and soul. With each sip of a nutrient-rich smoothie, you infuse your cells with vitality. With each colorful plate of vibrant fruits and vegetables, you celebrate the healing potential of nutrition. This is the art of nutritional healing, and it is a journey worth taking.
Let us begin.

Chapter References:

1. Sabaté, J., & Wien, M. (2010). Vegetarian diets and childhood obesity prevention. American Journal of Clinical Nutrition, 91(5), 1525S-1529S.
2. Tuso, P. J., Ismail, M. H., Ha, B. P., & Bartolotto, C. (2013). Nutritional update for physicians: Plant-based diets. The Permanente Journal, 17(2), 61-66.
3. Satija, A., Bhupathiraju, S. N., Spiegelman, D., Chiuve, S. E., Manson, J. E., Willett, W., ... & Hu, F. B. (2017). Healthful and unhealthful plant-based diets and the risk of coronary heart disease in US adults. Journal of the American College of Cardiology, 70(4), 411-422.

21

PART II: HEALING THROUGH FOOD

THE TRANSFORMATIVE POWER OF NUTRITION IN PREVENTING DISEASE

As we explore how to achieve healing through food, we delve deep into the profound ways in which nutrition can serve as a powerful tool for healing and preventing disease.

We explore the intricate connections between the foods we consume and their impact on our overall health, emphasizing the benefits of a high raw plant-based diet as a means of nourishing our bodies and promoting general well-being and even relief from certain chronic diseases.

Heart Health: Eating for a Strong Heart

The heart, an extraordinary organ at the center of our circulatory system, beats tirelessly, pumping blood to every cell in our body. Its well-being is paramount to our overall health, and our dietary choices play a pivotal role in nurturing and protecting this vital muscle.

Heart disease remains a leading cause of mortality worldwide, making it essential to understand the pivotal role of nutrition in promoting heart health. A high raw plant-based diet emerges as a cornerstone of cardiovascular wellness. This dietary approach emphasizes whole, unprocessed plant foods that are rich in fiber, antioxidants, and heart-protective nutrients.

In this section, we'll explore the intricate relationship between nutrition and heart health, highlighting the remarkable benefits of a high raw plant-based diet in promoting cardiovascular wellness. In particular, we will explain the science behind the impact of plant-based nutrition on cholesterol levels, blood pressure, and inflammation—key factors in heart health.

Learn how raw plant foods, such as leafy greens, berries, and nuts, can reduce the risk of heart disease and support a strong heart.

The Heart of the Matter

Heart disease, encompassing conditions such as coronary artery disease, heart failure, and hypertension, continues to be a global health concern. It remains one of the leading causes of morbidity and mortality, underscoring the urgency of adopting strategies to prevent and manage cardiovascular issues.

The Standard Western Diet and Heart Disease

The standard Western diet, characterized by its high intake of processed foods, saturated fats, cholesterol, and refined sugars, has been strongly linked to an increased risk of heart disease. This diet, often dubbed the "Standard American Diet" (SAD), is associated with elevated levels of LDL (low-density lipoprotein) cholesterol—the so-called "bad" cholesterol—increased blood pressure, inflammation, and a higher likelihood of obesity.

The detrimental effects of the SAD are exacerbated by its poor nutritional quality, leading to a cascade of health issues that strain the cardiovascular system. Fortunately, there is a better path—a path that emphasizes the healing power of nutrition and centers on the consumption of whole, raw plant-based foods.

A High Raw Plant-Based Diet and Heart Health

The concept of a high raw plant-based diet is rooted in the idea that humans are physiological frugivores, meaning that our bodies are naturally suited to thrive on a diet rich in fruits, vegetables, nuts, and seeds. This dietary approach aligns perfectly with the goal of heart health for several reasons.

- **Fiber and Cholesterol Management**: One of the key factors in heart health is the regulation of cholesterol levels. Excessive LDL cholesterol in the bloodstream can lead to the formation of plaques in the arteries, a process known as atherosclerosis. A high raw plant-based diet is naturally low in saturated fats and cholesterol while being rich in soluble fiber. Soluble fiber acts like a sponge, binding to cholesterol and helping to remove it from the body through the digestive system.

Foods such as oats, legumes, apples, and citrus fruits are excellent sources of soluble fiber, offering a natural way to lower LDL cholesterol levels.

- **Antioxidants and Inflammation Reduction**: Chronic inflammation plays a significant role in the development and progression of heart disease. Raw plant foods are abundant in antioxidants—compounds that neutralize harmful free radicals and reduce inflammation. Brightly colored fruits and vegetables like berries, spinach, and bell peppers are teeming with antioxidants, helping to protect the delicate lining of blood vessels and reduce the risk of inflammation-related heart issues.

- **Blood Pressure Regulation**: High blood pressure, or hypertension, is a common risk factor for heart disease. A diet rich in potassium, calcium, and magnesium—all prevalent in raw plant foods—can help regulate blood pressure. Leafy greens, bananas, and nuts are excellent sources of these minerals, contributing to healthy blood vessel function and reduced blood pressure.

- **Weight Management**: Maintaining a healthy weight is crucial for heart health. A high raw plant-based diet, with its emphasis on nutrient-dense, low-calorie foods, supports weight management. Fruits and vegetables are naturally low in calories but high in essential nutrients, making them a satisfying choice for those looking to shed excess pounds or maintain a healthy weight.

- **Endothelial Function**: The endothelium, the inner lining of blood vessels, plays a vital role in regulating blood flow and preventing clot formation. Consuming a high raw plant-based diet supports healthy endothelial function, ensuring that blood vessels remain flexible and responsive. This, in turn, reduces the risk of blood clots and plaque formation.

- **Healthy Fats**: While the diet is primarily plant-based, it also includes healthy fats from sources like nuts, seeds, and avocados. These fats are predominantly unsaturated, particularly monounsaturated and polyunsaturated fatty acids, which have been linked to heart health. They can help reduce levels of LDL cholesterol and support overall cardiovascular well-being.

- **Phytonutrients**: The rich spectrum of phytonutrients found in raw plant foods offers additional heart-protective benefits. For example, the flavonoids in berries and cocoa have been associated with improved blood vessel function, while the nitrate in leafy greens can help lower blood pressure. These natural compounds work in harmony to support cardiovascular wellness.

The Mediterranean Diet Connection and Heart Disease

It's worth noting that the principles of a high raw plant-based diet share many similarities with the Mediterranean diet, a dietary pattern renowned for its heart-healthy benefits.

The Mediterranean diet emphasizes fruits, vegetables, whole grains, nuts, seeds, and olive oil while limiting red meat and processed foods. Studies have consistently shown that adhering to a Mediterranean-style diet is associated with a reduced risk of heart disease, stroke, and other cardiovascular events.

What sets the high raw plant-based diet apart from that diet is its exclusive focus on plant foods in their natural, unprocessed state. By predominantly consuming raw fruits and vegetables and eliminating all animal products, individuals can further amplify the heart-protective properties of the Mediterranean dietary approach.

The Healing Potential of a High Raw Plant-Based Diet

The healing potential of a high raw plant-based diet for heart health is not just theoretical; it is supported by an ever-growing body of scientific research. Studies have demonstrated the benefits of plant-based nutrition in reducing the risk of heart disease and improving cardiovascular outcomes.

One landmark study, known as the Adventist Health Study-2, examined the dietary patterns of over 96,000 participants, including vegans, vegetarians, and omnivores. The research found that individuals following vegan diets had a significantly lower risk of heart disease, with a 42% reduced risk compared to those following an omnivorous diet. Vegetarians also had a reduced risk, with a 34% lower risk of heart disease.

Moreover, a review published in the Journal of the American College of Cardiology found that plant-based diets are associated with a lower risk of developing heart disease and a reduced risk of dying from heart-related causes.

These findings underscore the transformative power of a high raw plant-based diet in promoting heart health and reducing the risk of cardiovascular disease. By embracing this dietary approach, individuals can take proactive steps toward nurturing a strong, resilient heart and safeguarding their overall well-being.

Practical Tips for a Heart-Healthy High Raw Plant-Based Diet

Embracing a high raw plant-based diet for heart health can be both enjoyable and sustainable. Here are some practical tips to help you get started:

1. **Emphasize Fruits and Vegetables**: Make raw fruits and vegetables the cornerstone of your diet. Aim to fill half your plate with these vibrant foods at every meal. Experiment with a variety of colors and textures to maximize the range of nutrients and phytonutrients you consume.

2. **Incorporate Leafy Greens**: Leafy greens like kale, spinach, and Swiss chard are nutritional powerhouses. Include them in salads, smoothies, and green juices to boost your intake of vitamins, minerals, and antioxidants.

3. **Add Nuts and Seeds**: Incorporate a variety of nuts and seeds into your diet, such as almonds, walnuts, chia seeds, and flaxseeds. These nutrient-dense foods provide essential fats, protein, and fiber.

4. **Opt for Whole Grains**: Choose whole grains like quinoa, brown rice, and oats over refined grains. Whole grains are rich in fiber and provide sustained energy, making them a heart-healthy choice.

5. **Minimize Processed Foods**: Reduce or eliminate processed foods, which are often high in added sugars, unhealthy fats, and sodium. These foods can contribute to heart disease risk factors.

6. **Limit Salt Intake**: Excessive salt intake can raise blood pressure. Use herbs and spices to flavor your dishes, and reduce the use of table salt and processed foods high in sodium.

7. **Stay Hydrated**: Drink plenty of water and herbal teas to stay hydrated. Adequate hydration is essential for overall health and helps support healthy blood pressure.

8. **Moderate Fruit Consumption**: While fruits are a valuable part of a high raw plant-based diet, some individuals may need to monitor their fruit intake if they have specific dietary requirements, such as managing blood sugar levels. Consult with a healthcare professional or registered dietitian for personalized guidance.

9. **Practice Mindful Eating**: Pay attention to hunger and fullness cues, and eat mindfully. Eating slowly and savoring each bite can help prevent overeating.

10. **Consider Supplements**: Depending on individual needs, consider supplements like vitamin B12, vitamin D, and omega-3 fatty acids from walnuts or flax and hemp seeds to ensure optimal nutrition. Consult with a healthcare professional or nutritionist for personalized supplement recommendations.

By incorporating these principles into your daily life, you can harness the healing power of a high raw plant-based diet to support heart health, reduce the risk of heart disease, and promote overall well-being.

Section References:

1. Yokoyama, Y., Nishimura, K., Barnard, N. D., Takegami, M., Watanabe, M., Sekikawa, A., ... & Okamura, T. (2017). Vegetarian diets and blood pressure: A meta-analysis. JAMA Internal Medicine, 177(11), 1552-1560.

2. Satija, A., Bhupathiraju, S. N., Rimm, E. B., Spiegelman, D., Chiuve, S. E., Borgi, L., ... & Hu, F. B. (2017). Plant-based dietary patterns and incidence of type 2 diabetes in US men and women: Results from three prospective cohort studies. PLoS Medicine, 14(7), e1002039.

3. Ornish, D., Scherwitz, L. W., Billings, J. H., Brown, S. E., Gould, K. L., Merritt, T. A., ... & Brand, R. J. (1998). Intensive lifestyle changes for reversal of coronary heart disease. JAMA, 280(23), 2001-2007.

4. Esselstyn Jr, C. B., Gendy, G., Doyle, J., Golubic, M., & Roizen, M. F. (2014). A way to reverse CAD? Journal of Family Practice, 63(7), 356-364b.

5. Fraser, G. E. (2017). Vegetarian diets: what do we know of their effects on common chronic diseases? The American Journal of Clinical Nutrition, 100(suppl_1), 337S-343S.

6. Satija, A., Bhupathiraju, S. N., Spiegelman, D., Chiuve, S. E., Manson, J. E., Willett, W., & Rexrode, K. M. (2017). Healthful and unhealthful plant-based diets and the risk of coronary heart disease in US adults. Journal of the American College of Cardiology, 70(4), 411-422.

7. Tuso, P. J., Ismail, M. H., Ha, B. P., & Bartolotto, C. (2013). Nutritional update for physicians: Plant-based diets. The Permanente Journal, 17(2), 61-66.

Digestive Wellness: Nourishing Your Gut

The digestive system, often referred to as the "second brain," is a complex and integral part of our overall health. Its primary role is to break down the foods we eat into nutrients that our body can absorb and utilize.

A well-functioning digestive system is not only essential for nutrient absorption but also plays a central role in our immune function and overall well-being. Our digestive system is thus a central player in our health, influencing nutrient absorption, immune function, and overall vitality.

Optimal digestive wellness is achieved through a diet that promotes a balanced gut microbiota and supports efficient digestion. A high raw plant-based diet provides the fiber, prebiotics, and probiotics necessary for a thriving gut ecosystem.

In the sections below, we explore the importance of dietary fiber in maintaining regularity and preventing conditions such as constipation and diverticulitis. We will also discuss the profound influence of nutrition on digestive wellness, emphasizing the remarkable benefits of a high raw plant-based diet in nourishing your gut.

The Digestive System: A Symphony of Organs

Before delving into the impact of diet on digestive wellness, let's take a moment to appreciate the complexity of the digestive system. It consists of various organs, each with a specific role in the digestion and absorption of nutrients. These organs include:

- **Mouth**: Digestion begins in the mouth, where enzymes in saliva start breaking down carbohydrates.

- **Esophagus**: This muscular tube carries food from the mouth to the stomach through a process called peristalsis.

- **Stomach**: The stomach secretes gastric juices containing hydrochloric acid and enzymes that further break down food into a semi-liquid substance known as chyme.

- **Small Intestine**: The majority of nutrient absorption occurs in the small intestine, thanks to its large surface area. The pancreas and liver release enzymes and bile to aid digestion.

- **Large Intestine (Colon)**: The colon absorbs water and electrolytes from the remaining undigested food, forming feces for elimination.

- **Gut Microbiota**: Trillions of microorganisms, including bacteria, fungi, and viruses, reside in the gut. They play a critical role in digestion, nutrient absorption, and overall health.

This intricate system relies on the foods we consume to function optimally. A high raw plant-based diet aligns perfectly with the digestive system's needs, providing an abundance of fiber, prebiotics, and probiotics to support digestive wellness.

The Gut-Brain Connection

The gut and brain are intricately connected through the gut-brain axis, a complex communication network involving the central nervous system and the enteric nervous system in the gut. This connection allows the gut to influence mood, cognition, and behavior, while the brain can also affect gut function.

Emerging research has highlighted the role of the gut microbiota in this connection. The gut microbiota, often referred to as the "forgotten organ," plays a crucial role in maintaining a healthy gut-brain axis. An imbalance in the gut microbiota, known as dysbiosis, has been associated with various gastrointestinal disorders, such as irritable bowel syndrome (IBS), as well as neurological conditions, including anxiety and depression.

A high raw plant-based diet supports a healthy gut microbiota by providing an abundance of fiber, which serves as a prebiotic—a substance that feeds beneficial gut bacteria. Raw plant foods also contain phytonutrients that have been linked to improved mood and cognitive function, further enhancing the gut-brain connection.

Fiber and Regularity

One of the key benefits of a high raw plant-based diet for digestive wellness is its rich fiber content. Dietary fiber is the indigestible part of plant foods that adds bulk to the diet and facilitates regular bowel movements. There are two main types of dietary fiber:

- **Soluble Fiber**: This type of fiber dissolves in water and forms a gel-like substance in the digestive tract. It can help lower cholesterol levels and stabilize blood sugar levels. Foods rich in soluble fiber include oats, legumes, apples, and citrus fruits.

- **Insoluble Fiber**: Insoluble fiber does not dissolve in water and adds bulk to stool, promoting regular bowel movements. It can be found in foods like whole grains, nuts, seeds, and vegetables.

A high raw plant-based diet is abundant in both types of fiber, ensuring that the digestive system remains healthy and efficient. Adequate fiber intake can prevent constipation, diverticulitis, and other gastrointestinal issues while supporting overall digestive wellness.

Prebiotics and Probiotics

In addition to fiber, raw plant foods like sauerkraut, kimchi, and fermented plant-based yogurts contribute to a healthy gut microbiota, bolstering our immune system and reducing the risk of gastrointestinal disorders. Raw plant foods are also rich in prebiotics and probiotics—two essential components for a healthy gut microbiota.

Prebiotics are non-digestible fibers that serve as food for beneficial gut bacteria. They promote the growth and activity of these beneficial microbes, enhancing gut health. Common prebiotic-rich foods in a high raw plant-based diet include garlic, onions, leeks, and Jerusalem artichokes.

Probiotics are live microorganisms that provide health benefits when consumed in adequate amounts. They can be found in fermented foods like sauerkraut, kimchi, plant-based yogurts, and kefir. Probiotics help maintain a balanced gut microbiota and support immune function.

A high raw plant-based diet naturally incorporates these gut-friendly components, promoting a thriving gut microbiota and digestive wellness.

Inflammation Reduction

Chronic inflammation is a contributing factor to many digestive disorders, including inflammatory bowel disease (IBD) and IBS. A high raw plant-based diet is inherently anti-inflammatory due to its rich array of antioxidants and phytonutrients.

These compounds combat oxidative stress and inflammation, protecting the gut lining from damage and reducing the risk of inflammation-related digestive issues. Fruits and vegetables like berries, leafy greens, and cruciferous vegetables are particularly potent sources of anti-inflammatory phytonutrients.

Supporting a Healthy Gut Microbiota

The gut microbiota is a diverse community of microorganisms residing in the digestive tract. It plays a fundamental role in nutrient absorption, immune function, and overall health. A high raw plant-based diet positively influences the gut microbiota in several ways:

- **Diversity**: Raw plant foods contain a wide range of fibers and phytonutrients that nourish different types of gut bacteria, promoting a diverse microbiota.
- **Fermentable Substrates**: The fiber in raw plant foods serves as a substrate for fermentation by beneficial gut bacteria. This fermentation process produces short-chain fatty acids (SCFAs), which contribute to gut health and have anti-inflammatory properties.
- **Bacterial Balance**: A high raw plant-based diet supports a balanced ratio of beneficial bacteria to harmful bacteria in the gut, reducing the risk of dysbiosis and gastrointestinal issues.

Gut Health and Disease Prevention

The importance of digestive wellness extends beyond daily comfort—it plays a crucial role in disease prevention. A healthy gut can reduce the risk of various gastrointestinal conditions, including:

Irritable Bowel Syndrome (IBS): A high raw plant-based diet can alleviate symptoms of IBS, such as bloating, abdominal pain, and irregular bowel movements, by providing soluble fiber and minimizing irritants found in processed foods.

Inflammatory Bowel Disease (IBD): While dietary triggers for IBD are complex and multifactorial, a high raw plant-based diet may help reduce inflammation and promote gut healing.

Colorectal Cancer: A diet rich in raw plant foods has been associated with a reduced risk of colorectal cancer due to its high fiber content and the presence of antioxidants that combat free radicals.

Gastroesophageal Reflux Disease (GERD): By avoiding acidic and spicy foods commonly associated with GERD, a high raw plant-based diet may help alleviate symptoms and promote digestive comfort.

Practical Tips for Nourishing Your Gut with a High Raw Plant-Based

Diet

By embracing a high raw plant-based diet and implementing the following practical tips, you can nourish your gut, support digestive wellness, and reduce the risk of gastrointestinal issues.

1. **Gradual Transition**: If you're new to a high raw plant-based diet, consider a gradual transition. Begin by incorporating more raw fruits and vegetables into your meals and snacks, increasing the raw component over time.
2. **Hydration**: Stay well-hydrated by drinking water and herbal teas. Hydration is essential for healthy digestion.
3. **Chew Thoroughly**: Take your time to chew your food thoroughly. This aids in the mechanical breakdown of food and promotes proper digestion.
4. **Fermented Foods**: Include fermented foods like sauerkraut, kimchi, and plant-based yogurts in your diet to introduce beneficial probiotics.
5. **Variety**: Aim for a diverse range of fruits and vegetables to provide your gut microbiota with a wide array of nutrients and fibers.
6. **Limit Processed Foods**: Minimize processed foods, which can disrupt gut health due to their often low fiber content and high levels of additives.
7. **Mindful Eating**: Practice mindful eating to reduce stress and support optimal digestion. Avoid overeating and consume meals in a relaxed environment.
8. **Supplements**: Consider probiotic supplements, especially if you have a history of gastrointestinal issues or if you're in the process of transitioning to a high raw plant-based diet.
9. **Seek Professional Guidance**: If you have specific digestive concerns or conditions, consult with a healthcare professional or registered dietitian for personalized advice and guidance.

Keep in mind that your gut is not only the center of your digestive system but also a vital component of your overall health and well-being.

Section References:

1. Rinninella, E., Raoul, P., Cintoni, M., Franceschi, F., Miggiano, G. A. D., Gasbarrini, A., & Mele, M. C. (2019). What is the healthy gut microbiota composition? A changing ecosystem across age, environment, diet, and diseases. Microorganisms, 7(1), 14.
2. Turnbaugh, P. J., Ley, R. E., Hamady, M., Fraser-Liggett, C. M.,

Knight, R., & Gordon, J. I. (2007). The human microbiome project. Nature, 449(7164), 804-810.

3. Holscher, H. D. (2017). Dietary fiber and prebiotics and the gastrointestinal microbiota. Gut Microbes, 8(2), 172-184.

4. Cani, P. D., & Knauf, C. (2016). How gut microbes talk to organs: The role of endocrine and nervous routes. Molecular Metabolism, 5(9), 743-752.

5. Kelly, J. R., Kennedy, P. J., Cryan, J. F., Dinan, T. G., Clarke, G., & Hyland, N. P. (2015). Breaking down the barriers: the gut microbiome, intestinal permeability and stress-related psychiatric disorders. Frontiers in Cellular Neuroscience, 9, 392.

6. Mayer, E. A., Knight, R., Mazmanian, S. K., Cryan, J. F., & Tillisch, K. (2014). Gut microbes and the brain: paradigm shift in neuroscience. Journal of Neuroscience, 34(46), 15490-15496.

7. Rieder, R., Wisniewski, P. J., Alderman, B. L., & Campbell, S. C. (2017). Microbes and mental health: A review. Brain, Behavior, and Immunity, 66, 9-17.

8. O'Keefe, S. J. D., Li, J. V., Lahti, L., Ou, J., Carbonero, F., Mohammed, K., ... & Gill, B. D. (2015). Fat, fibre and cancer risk in African Americans and rural Africans. Nature Communications, 6, 6342.

9. De Filippis, F., Pellegrini, N., Vannini, L., Jeffery, I. B., La Storia, A., Laghi, L., ... & Ercolini, D. (2016). High-level adherence to a Mediterranean diet beneficially impacts the gut microbiota and associated metabolome. Gut, 65(11), 1812-1821.

Brain Health: Food for Thought

The human brain, often regarded as the body's command center, is a marvel of complexity and functionality. Its health and performance are influenced by a myriad of factors, and one of the most profound is the food we consume.

In fact, nutrition plays a pivotal role in cognitive function, mood regulation, and the prevention of neurodegenerative diseases. A high raw plant-based diet is a brain-boosting powerhouse, providing essential nutrients such as omega-3 fatty acids, antioxidants, and phytonutrients that support mental clarity and emotional well-being.

In this section, we'll explore the intricate relationship between nutrition and brain health, highlighting the exceptional benefits of a high raw plant-based diet in nourishing and protecting this vital organ.

Dive into the science of brain-boosting foods, including blueberries, walnuts, and leafy greens as you learn how a diet rich in raw plant foods can reduce the risk of cognitive decline and support a vibrant, resilient mind.

The Brain: A Remarkable Organ

The brain is an intricate network of billions of neurons that communicate with each other through electrical and chemical signals. It controls our thoughts, emotions, movements, and physiological functions, making it the epicenter of our consciousness and well-being.

Brain health is not solely about preventing neurological disorders; it also encompasses optimizing cognitive function, supporting emotional well-being, and preserving memory as we age. The foods we eat play a pivotal role in achieving these objectives.

Nutrition and Cognitive Function

Cognitive function encompasses a wide range of mental processes, including memory, attention, problem-solving, and creativity. These processes rely on the brain's ability to form and maintain neural connections, a function influenced by the availability of essential nutrients.

A high raw plant-based diet provides a wealth of these essential nutrients, promoting cognitive function in several ways:

- **Antioxidants**: Raw plant foods are rich in antioxidants, which combat oxidative stress and inflammation in the brain. Oxidative stress can damage brain cells and impair cognitive function. Antioxidants, found in abundance in fruits and vegetables like berries, spinach, and kale, protect the brain from this damage.

- **Omega-3 Fatty Acids**: Essential for brain health, omega-3 fatty acids are primarily found in foods like flaxseeds, hemp seeds, chia seeds, and walnuts. These fatty acids support the structure and function of brain cell membranes and have been linked to improved cognitive function and a reduced risk of cognitive decline.

- **Phytonutrients**: Phytonutrients in raw plant foods have been shown to enhance cognitive function. For instance, flavonoids, found in berries and dark chocolate, have been associated with better memory and learning.

- **B Vitamins**: B vitamins, particularly folate, vitamin B6, and vitamin B12, are essential for brain health. A deficiency in these vitamins can lead to cognitive impairment. Raw plant foods like leafy greens, legumes, and fortified plant-based foods can provide these vital nutrients.

- **Carotenoids**: Carotenoids, found in foods like carrots, sweet potatoes, and dark leafy greens, have been linked to improved cognitive performance and a reduced risk of cognitive decline.

- **Minerals**: Minerals like magnesium and zinc, abundant in raw plant foods, are crucial for neuronal function and the transmission of nerve signals.

- **Hydration**: Proper hydration is essential for optimal brain function. Water is involved in various neurological processes, including the transmission of electrical signals.

The Gut-Brain Connection

Emerging research has unveiled the profound connection between the gut and the brain, often referred to as the gut-brain axis. This bidirectional communication system influences not only cognitive function but also mood and emotional well-being.

A high raw plant-based diet supports a healthy gut microbiota, which, in turn, positively impacts the gut-brain axis. The gut microbiota produces neurotransmitters like serotonin, which plays a crucial role in regulating mood. A balanced and diverse gut microbiota is essential for emotional well-being and may contribute to reduced symptoms of depression and anxiety.

Furthermore, the gut microbiota influences inflammation and immune function, both of which are implicated in neurological disorders like Alzheimer's disease and Parkinson's disease. By nourishing the gut microbiota with a high raw plant-based diet, individuals can help protect their brain from inflammation and support cognitive health.

Diet and Neurological Disorders

While diet alone cannot guarantee immunity from neurological disorders, it can significantly reduce the risk and slow their progression. Several neurological conditions are influenced by diet, including:

- **Alzheimer's Disease**: A diet rich in antioxidants and omega-3 fatty acids, as found in raw plant foods, may reduce the risk of Alzheimer's disease and slow cognitive decline.
- **Parkinson's Disease**: Antioxidants and anti-inflammatory compounds in raw plant foods may protect against oxidative stress and inflammation, potentially reducing the risk of Parkinson's disease.
- **Stroke**: A diet high in fruits and vegetables has been associated with a reduced risk of stroke due to its ability to support healthy blood vessels and reduce inflammation.
- **Multiple Sclerosis (MS)**: Omega-3 fatty acids, found in abundance in a high raw plant-based diet, have been studied for their potential to reduce the risk of MS and mitigate symptoms.
- **Depression and Anxiety**: Plant-based diets, particularly those rich in fruits and vegetables, have been associated with a lower risk of depression and anxiety. The gut-brain axis plays a key role in this relationship.
- **Cognitive Decline**: Nutrient-dense diets that support brain health may slow the progression of age-related cognitive decline and neurodegenerative diseases.

The Mediterranean Diet Connection

We have already mentioned that the Mediterranean diet, known for its health benefits, shares many principles and benefits with a high raw plant-based diet. It emphasizes fruits, vegetables, whole grains, nuts, seeds, and olive oil while minimizing red meat and processed foods.

Research has consistently shown that adhering to a Mediterranean-style diet is associated with improved cognitive function and a reduced risk of cognitive decline.

What sets the high raw plant-based diet apart is its exclusive focus on raw plant foods in their natural state which contains vital nutrients that improves the immune system and energy levels, as well as vascular health.

By predominantly consuming fruits, vegetables, nuts, and seeds in their raw form, individuals can maximize the brain-boosting potential of this dietary approach.

Practical Tips for Nourishing Your Brain with a High Raw Plant-Based Diet

If you want to enjoy the benefits of a healthy brain, then you can incorporate the following tips into your dietary plan.

1. **Colorful Variety**: Aim to consume a wide array of colorful fruits and vegetables. Different colors often indicate unique phytonutrient profiles, so variety is key for optimal brain health.

2. **Omega-3 Rich Foods**: Include sources of omega-3 fatty acids, such as flaxseeds, chia seeds, hemp seeds and walnuts, in your daily diet.

3. **Antioxidant Power**: Incorporate antioxidant-rich foods like berries, dark leafy greens, and nuts to combat oxidative stress in the brain.

4. **Hydration**: Stay well-hydrated to support overall brain function. Herbal teas and water are excellent choices.

5. **Limit Processed Foods**: Minimize processed foods, refined sugars, and artificial additives, which can contribute to inflammation and negatively impact cognitive health.

6. **Mindful Eating**: Practice mindful eating to savor and appreciate the flavors and textures of your food. It promotes a positive relationship with food and can reduce overeating.

7. **Balanced Nutrient Intake**: Ensure a balanced intake of essential nutrients, including B vitamins, minerals, and phytonutrients, by eating a variety of raw plant foods.

8. **Consult with a Registered Dietitian:** If you have specific dietary concerns or health conditions, consider consulting with a registered dietitian to create a personalized nutrition plan.

By adopting these brain health promoting nutritional practices and embracing a high raw plant-based diet, you can provide your brain with the nourishment it needs to thrive, support cognitive function, and reduce the risk of neurological disorders. Food for thought indeed!

Section References:

1. Fotuhi, M., Mohassel, P., & Yaffe, K. (2009). Fish consumption, long-chain omega-3 fatty acids, and risk of cognitive decline or Alzheimer disease: a complex association. Nature Clinical Practice Neurology, 5(3), 140-152.
2. Gómez-Pinilla, F. (2008). Brain foods: the effects of nutrients on brain function. Nature Reviews Neuroscience, 9(7), 568-578.
3. Morris, M. C., Tangney, C. C., Wang, Y., Sacks, F. M., Bennett, D. A., & Aggarwal, N. T. (2015). MIND diet associated with reduced incidence of Alzheimer's disease. Alzheimer's & Dementia, 11(9), 1007-1014.
4. Lourida, I., Soni, M., Thompson-Coon, J., Purandare, N., Lang, I. A., Ukoumunne, O. C., & Llewellyn, D. J. (2013). Mediterranean diet, cognitive function, and dementia: a systematic review. Epidemiology, 24(4), 479-489.
5. Parletta, N., Zarnowiecki, D., Cho, J., Wilson, A., Bogomolova, S., Villani, A., ... & O'Dea, K. (2017). A Mediterranean-style dietary intervention supplemented with fish oil improves diet quality and mental health in people with depression: A randomized controlled trial (HELFIMED). Nutritional Neuroscience, 22(7), 474-487.
6. Jacka, F. N., O'Neil, A., Opie, R., Itsiopoulos, C., Cotton, S., Mohebbi, M., ... & Berk, M. (2017). A randomised controlled trial of dietary improvement for adults with major depression (the 'SMILES' trial). BMC Medicine, 15(1), 23.
7. Berr, C., Portet, F., Carriere, I., Akbaraly, T. N., Feart, C., Gourlet, V., ... & Ritchie, K. (2009). Olive oil and cognition: results from the Three-City Study. Dementia and Geriatric Cognitive Disorders, 28(4), 357-364.
8. Devore, E. E., Kang, J. H., Breteler, M. M., & Grodstein, F. (2012). Dietary intakes of berries and flavonoids in relation to cognitive decline. Annals of Neurology, 72(1), 135-143.

Immune Support: Boosting Your Defenses

The immune system serves as our body's defense against pathogens, infections and diseases, making it crucial to support its function through good nutrition. A strong immune system not only helps us fend off infections but also plays a role in preventing chronic diseases.

Operating as a complex network of cells, tissues and organs working in unison to protect us from harm, a robust and well-functioning immune system is vital for overall health and well-being. A high raw plant-based diet is a natural ally in fortifying our immune system's defenses.

In this section, we will delve into the profound impact of nutrition on immune support, emphasizing the remarkable benefits of a high raw plant-based diet in bolstering your body's defense responses. We will explore the immune-boosting properties of foods like citrus fruits, garlic, and mushrooms, which are rich in vitamins, minerals, and phytonutrients that enhance immune function.

Discover how raw plant foods can help reduce the duration and severity of illnesses and provide the immune support needed to thrive.

The Immune System: Our Shield Against Illness

The immune system's primary mission is to identify and neutralize harmful invaders, such as viruses, bacteria, and other pathogens. It does so through a two-pronged approach of innate and adaptive immunity.

Innate immunity is the body's first line of defense, providing immediate but non-specific protection. Innate immunity includes physical barriers like the skin, as well as immune cells like neutrophils and macrophages that patrol the body and engulf foreign invaders.

In contrast, adaptive immunity is a more specific and targeted response. It involves the production of antibodies and specialized immune cells, like T cells and B cells, which are tailored to recognize and eliminate specific pathogens. This arm of the immune system forms the basis of immunity after vaccination.

A well-balanced and properly nourished immune system is essential for preventing infections, reducing the severity and duration of illnesses, and even playing a role in preventing chronic diseases.

Nutrition and Immune Function

The foods we consume have a profound influence on the immune system's strength and efficacy. Proper nutrition provides the building blocks and energy required for immune cells to function optimally. A high raw plant-based diet aligns perfectly with these needs, offering a rich array of nutrients that support immune function:

1. **Vitamins and Minerals**: Essential vitamins and minerals, including vitamin C, vitamin D, vitamin E, zinc, selenium, and iron, are integral to immune health. These nutrients act as cofactors for various immune processes and play a role in antibody production, cell signaling, and immune cell activation.

2. **Antioxidants**: Raw plant foods are packed with antioxidants, such as flavonoids, carotenoids, and polyphenols, which help combat oxidative stress and inflammation, both of which can weaken the immune system.

3. **Fiber**: Fiber, abundant in fruits, vegetables, and whole grains, supports a healthy gut microbiota. A balanced gut microbiome is essential for immune function, as it helps regulate the immune response and protect against infections.

4. **Phytonutrients**: Phytonutrients are compounds found exclusively in plant-based foods. They have been linked to enhanced immune function, reduced inflammation, and improved overall health. For example, the compound allicin in garlic has antimicrobial properties, while the curcumin in turmeric exhibits anti-inflammatory and antioxidant effects.

5. **Omega-3 Fatty Acids**: Omega-3 fatty acids, primarily found in flaxseeds, hemp seeds, chia seeds, and walnuts, have anti-inflammatory properties that support immune function. They help modulate the immune response and reduce inflammation.

6. **Probiotics**: Fermented foods, a staple in a high raw plant-based diet, contain probiotics that contribute to a healthy gut microbiota. A balanced gut microbiome positively impacts immune function by promoting a balanced inflammatory response and aiding in pathogen defense.

7. **Hydration**: Proper hydration is essential for all bodily functions, including immune responses. Water helps transport nutrients and immune cells throughout the body, ensuring they can reach their destinations effectively.

A High Raw Plant-Based Diet and Immunity

A high raw plant-based diet provides an exceptional foundation for immune support due to its nutrient density and anti-inflammatory properties. Here's how it contributes to a robust immune system:

- **Vitamin C**: Raw fruits, such as citrus fruits, strawberries and other berries, tomatoes, and bell peppers, are excellent sources of vitamin C. This vitamin plays a central role in immune function by promoting the production and function of immune cells, such as white blood cells and lymphocytes.

- **B Vitamins**: Raw plant foods contribute essential B vitamins that boost your energy level. These ephemeral vitamins are destroyed in cooked food.

- **Vitamin D**: While vitamin D is less abundant in raw plant foods, it can be obtained from sun exposure and fortified plant-based sources like fortified plant-based milk and cereals. Vitamin D supports immune function by enhancing the body's defense mechanisms.

- **Zinc**: Raw nuts and seeds, such as pumpkin seeds and cashews, are rich in zinc, a mineral that supports immune cell development and function. A zinc deficiency can impair your immune system's responses.

- **Antioxidants**: The antioxidant-rich nature of raw plant foods helps protect immune cells from damage caused by free radicals, ensuring they can function optimally.

- **Fiber and Gut Health**: A high raw plant-based diet supports a diverse and balanced gut microbiota. This balance is essential for immune health, as a significant portion of immune cells resides in the gut-associated lymphoid tissue (GALT).

- **Hydration**: Staying well-hydrated ensures that immune cells can circulate efficiently throughout the body and reach infection sites.

The Gut Microbiota and Immunity

The gut microbiota, composed of trillions of microorganisms residing in the digestive tract, plays a pivotal role in immune function. A balanced and diverse gut microbiome is associated with better immune responses, while dysbiosis (an imbalance) can lead to immune dysregulation.

A high raw plant-based diet supports gut health in several ways. First of all, raw plant foods are rich in fiber, which serves as a prebiotic—a substance that feeds beneficial gut bacteria. A diet high in fiber promotes the growth of beneficial bacteria that support immune function.

Secondly, the fiber in raw plant foods serves as a fermentable substrate for beneficial gut bacteria. This fermentation process produces short-chain fatty acids (SCFAs), which have immune-enhancing properties.

The diversity of plant-based foods in a high raw diet also promotes a diverse gut microbiota, which is associated with enhanced immune resilience.

Finally, fermented plant foods like sauerkraut, kimchi, and plant-based yogurts contain probiotics that contribute to a healthy gut microbiota, further supporting immune system health.

Immune Health and Disease Prevention

A robust immune system is not only essential for fighting infections but also plays a pivotal role in preventing chronic diseases. Here are some ways in which a high raw plant-based diet can contribute to disease prevention through immune support:

1. **Infectious Diseases**: A strong immune system is your first line of defense against infectious diseases. Proper nutrition and a high raw plant-based diet can help reduce the risk of infections and their complications.

2. **Chronic Inflammatory Diseases**: Chronic inflammation is a common thread in many chronic diseases, including heart disease, diabetes, and cancer. A diet rich in anti-inflammatory raw plant foods can help modulate inflammation and reduce the risk of these conditions.

3. **Autoimmune Diseases**: Autoimmune diseases occur when the immune system mistakenly targets the body's own tissues. While

diet alone cannot cure autoimmune diseases, a high raw plant-based diet can help reduce inflammation and support overall immune health.

4. **Cancer**: A well-functioning immune system can identify and destroy cancer cells. Phytonutrients and antioxidants in raw plant foods support the immune system's cancer-fighting capabilities.

Practical Tips for Immune Support with a High Raw Plant-Based Diet

If you want to enjoy the benefits of a healthy immune system, then you can incorporate the following tips into your dietary plan.

1. **Diverse Diet**: Consume a wide variety of raw fruits, leafy greens, vegetables, nuts, seeds, and legumes to ensure you get a broad spectrum of nutrients and phytonutrients.

2. **Hydration**: Stay well-hydrated with water and herbal teas to support immune cell circulation.

3. **Probiotics**: Include some fermented foods like sauerkraut, kimchi, and plant-based yogurts in your diet periodically to introduce and maintain beneficial probiotics in your digestive system.

4. **Vitamin D**: If needed, consider vitamin D supplements or fortified plant-based foods, especially if you have limited sun exposure.

5. **Stress Management**: Chronic stress can weaken the immune system. Practice stress-reduction techniques such as meditation, yoga, and deep breathing.

6. **Regular Physical Activity**: Engage in regular physical activity to enhance immune function and overall health.

7. **Adequate Sleep**: Ensure you get sufficient quality sleep, as sleep is essential for immune cell regeneration.

8. **Whole Foods**: Choose whole, minimally processed foods to maximize nutrient intake and minimize exposure to additives and preservatives.

By adopting these practices and embracing a high raw plant-based diet, you can fortify your immune system, reduce the risk of infections and chronic diseases, and enjoy enhanced overall well-being. Remember, your immune system is your body's natural defender, so be sure to empower it with the nutrition it needs to thrive.

Section References:

1. Gombart, A. F., Pierre, A., & Maggini, S. (2020). A review of micronutrients and the immune system-working in harmony to reduce the risk of infection. Nutrients, 12(1), 236.
2. Calder, P. C., Carr, A. C., Gombart, A. F., & Eggersdorfer, M. (2020). Optimal nutritional status for a well-functioning immune system is an important factor to protect against viral infections. Nutrients, 12(4), 1181.
3. Maggini, S., Pierre, A., & Calder, P. C. (2018). Immune function and micronutrient requirements change over the life course. Nutrients, 10(10), 1531.
4. Thorburn, A. N., Macia, L., & Mackay, C. R. (2014). Diet, metabolites, and "western-lifestyle" inflammatory diseases. Immunity, 40(6), 833-842.
5. Wu, D., & Lewis, E. D. (2019). Paeoniflorin: a monomer from traditional Chinese medical herb ameliorates lipid induced inflammation in L02 and Kupffer cells. Lipids in Health and Disease, 18(1), 1-11.
6. Gibson, G. R., Hutkins, R., Sanders, M. E., Prescott, S. L., Reimer, R. A., Salminen, S. J., ... & Reid, G. (2017). Expert consensus document: The International Scientific Association for Probiotics and Prebiotics (ISAPP) consensus statement on the definition and scope of prebiotics. Nature Reviews Gastroenterology & Hepatology, 14(8), 491-502.
7. Round, J. L., & Mazmanian, S. K. (2009). The gut microbiota shapes intestinal immune responses during health and disease. Nature Reviews Immunology, 9(5), 313-323.
8. Calder, P. C. (2013). Omega-3 fatty acids and inflammatory processes: from molecules to man. Biochemical Society Transactions, 41(6), 1105-1115.
9. Schwingshackl, L., Schwedhelm, C., Galbete, C., & Hoffmann, G. (2017). Adherence to Mediterranean diet and risk of cancer: an updated systematic review and meta-analysis. Nutrients, 9(10), 1063.

Weight Management: Finding Balance

Weight management is a concern for many, and achieving and maintaining a healthy weight is a cornerstone of overall well-being. Weight management involves striking a balance between the calories you consume and the calories your body expends. It's not just about aesthetics; it's also about optimizing health and reducing the risk of chronic diseases.

A high raw plant-based diet offers a unique approach to weight wellness, focusing on natural, nutrient-dense foods that support satiety and healthy metabolism.

In this section, we delve into the science of weight management, exploring how a high raw plant-based diet promotes a healthy body composition and can be a powerful tool for weight management, promoting both physical health and vitality.

You will learn about the role of dietary fiber in promoting fullness and reducing overeating, as well as the benefits of whole grains, legumes, and nuts in supporting a balanced weight. You'll also discover how raw plant foods contribute to a vibrant, active lifestyle that supports weight wellness.

The Significance of Healthy Weight Management

Maintaining a healthy weight is essential for various reasons, including:

- **Reduced Risk of Chronic Diseases**: Excess body weight is a major risk factor for chronic conditions such as heart disease, type 2 diabetes, hypertension, and certain cancers. Achieving and maintaining a healthy weight can significantly reduce the risk of developing these diseases.

- **Improved Cardiovascular Health**: Weight management can lower the risk of cardiovascular problems such as high blood pressure, high cholesterol, and atherosclerosis. It also reduces the strain on the heart and improves overall cardiovascular function.

- **Enhanced Physical Function**: Maintaining a healthy weight supports physical function and mobility. It can help prevent musculoskeletal issues, joint pain, and injuries.

- **Better Mental Health**: A healthy weight is associated with improved mental health, self-esteem, and body image. It can reduce the risk of conditions like depression and anxiety.

- **Quality of Life**: Healthy weight management contributes to an overall improved quality of life, allowing individuals to engage in daily activities with ease and enjoy a higher level of vitality.

The Role of Diet in Weight Management

Diet plays a central role in weight management. The foods you choose to consume can either support or hinder your efforts to achieve and maintain a healthy weight. A high raw plant-based diet offers distinct advantages in this regard, including the following:

- **Low Caloric Density**: Raw plant foods are generally lower in calories and higher in water and fiber content compared to processed and animal-based foods. This low caloric density makes it easier to control calorie intake while still enjoying satisfying meals.

- **Fiber Content**: Fiber-rich foods like fruits, leafy greens, vegetables, whole grains, and legumes are a hallmark of a high raw plant-based diet. Dietary fiber promotes satiety, reducing the likelihood of overeating and supporting weight management.

- **Nutrient Density**: Raw plant foods are nutrient powerhouses, providing essential vitamins, minerals, and phytonutrients without excess calories. This nutrient density ensures that your body receives vital nutrients while managing weight effectively.

- **Reduction in Processed Foods**: A high raw plant-based diet naturally reduces the consumption of processed foods, which are often calorie-dense and nutrient-poor. Minimizing processed foods can help control calorie intake.

- **Improved Insulin Sensitivity**: Some studies suggest that a plant-based diet may improve insulin sensitivity, which can aid in weight management by regulating blood sugar levels and reducing fat storage.

- **Enhanced Gut Health**: A diet rich in raw plant foods supports a balanced gut microbiota, which may play a role in weight regulation. A healthy gut microbiome can improve nutrient absorption and influence metabolic processes.

- **Anti-Inflammatory Effects**: Chronic inflammation is associated with weight gain and obesity. The anti-inflammatory nature of raw plant foods may help mitigate this risk.

Weight Management with a High Raw Plant-Based Diet

A high raw plant-based diet aligns well with the principles of weight management. Here's how it can aid in achieving and maintaining a healthy weight:

- **Calorie Control**: Raw plant foods are typically lower in calories, allowing individuals to consume satisfying portions without excessive calorie intake. This can promote weight loss when needed or help maintain a healthy weight.

- **Satiety**: The high fiber content of raw plant foods enhances feelings of fullness and satiety, reducing the temptation to overeat or snack on calorie-dense foods.

- **Balanced Macronutrients**: A high raw plant-based diet provides a balanced ratio of macronutrients, including carbohydrates, healthy fats, and plant-based proteins. This balance supports overall health and energy while managing weight.

- **Natural Hydration**: Many raw plant foods, such as fruits and vegetables, have a high water content, contributing to hydration. Proper hydration can reduce the likelihood of mistaking thirst for hunger.

- **Whole Foods**: Whole, minimally processed and fresh raw foods are a fundamental component of a high raw plant-based diet. These foods are generally more filling and nutrient-dense than their processed counterparts.

- **Sustainable Approach**: A high raw plant-based diet is sustainable over the long term, making it a practical choice for those aiming to maintain a healthy weight throughout their lives.

- **Metabolic Benefits**: Some research suggests that plant-based diets can have metabolic benefits, such as improved insulin sensitivity, which may aid in weight management.

Intermittent Fasting

Intermittent fasting (IF) is an eating pattern that cycles between periods of fasting and eating and can assist in weight management. This technique does not specify which foods you should eat but rather when you should eat them.

Several different ways to practice intermittent fasting exist, but they all involve alternating periods of fasting and eating. Some popular methods include:

- **The 16/8 Method:** This involves skipping breakfast and restricting your daily eating period to 8 hours, such as 1–9 p.m. Then you would fast for 16 hours in between.

- **Eat-Stop-Eat:** This involves fasting for 24 hours, once or twice a week, for example by not eating from dinner one day until dinner the next day.

- **The 5:2 Diet:** With this method, you consume only 500–600 calories on two nonconsecutive days of the week, but eat normally the other 5 days.

Intermittent fasting helps the body burn fat, so it is currently popular for weight loss and has been shown to have powerful effects on the body and brain. It may even help you live longer since caloric restriction tends to increase life span.

With that noted, it's important to consider one's health conditions, social and economic supports, culture, and more in order to decide if following an intermittent fasting regimen is appropriate.

Since intermittent fasting may not be suitable for everyone, if you have any underlying health conditions or concerns, it's best to consult with a healthcare professional before starting a dietary regimen that includes intermittent fasting.

Weight Adjustment Tips

If you wish to lose weight, then focus more on consuming a balanced amount of fruits and greens, keeping other foods to less than 10% of your overall diet. Once your ideal weight has been achieved, then you can start to add more plant-derived fat sources like avocadoes, nuts, nut butters, seeds and coconut to stabilize your weight.

Keep in mind that coconut contains a substantial amount of saturated fat, so that food may not suit someone seeking to heal from vascular disease. Also, techniques like intermittent fasting can help burn fat and reduce fat mass as a percentage of body weight.

On the other hand, if you wish to gain weight, then you can increase your caloric intake and add more of the above mentioned fat sources to your diet since they provide extra calories and insulin resistance that can help deposit stores of fat on your body. You will also want to avoid intermittent fasting.

Finally, those wishing to gain muscle, can embark on an exercise plan and include some high protein sources like nuts and seeds, as well as sprouted garbanzo beans, mung beans and lentils, until they have achieved their desired body-building objective. Using techniques like intermittent fasting can also help increase muscle mass as a percentage of body weight.

Practical Tips for Weight Management with a High Raw Plant-Based Diet

If you want to enjoy the weight management benefits of a high raw plant-based diet, then you can incorporate the following tips into your dietary plan.

1. **Balanced Meals**: Create balanced meals that incorporate a variety of raw fruits, leafy greens, vegetables, nuts, seeds, whole grains, and legumes to ensure a comprehensive intake of nutrients.

2. **Portion Control**: While raw plant foods are lower in calories, portion control is still important. Be mindful of portion sizes to avoid excessive calorie intake.

3. **Hydration**: Ensure you stay well-hydrated by drinking water and herbal teas throughout the day. Proper hydration can reduce the urge to snack unnecessarily.

4. **Physical Activity**: Combine a high raw plant-based diet with regular physical activity for optimal weight management and overall health.

5. **Mindful Eating**: Practice mindful eating by paying attention to your body's hunger and fullness cues. Avoid eating out of boredom or stress.

6. **Healthy Fats**: Include low to moderate amounts of sources of healthy fats like avocados, nuts, and seeds in your diet for satiety and overall nutritional balance.

7. **Whole Grains**: Choose whole grains over refined grains for sustained energy and enhanced satiety.

8. **Consult with a Registered Dietitian**: If you have specific weight management goals or dietary concerns, consider consulting with a registered dietitian for personalized guidance.

By embracing a high raw plant-based diet and following these practical tips, you can take proactive steps toward achieving and maintaining a healthy weight. This dietary approach not only supports weight management but also contributes to overall health, vitality, and longevity.

Section References:

1. Turner-McGrievy, G. M., & Wirth, M. D. (2017). Comparison of plant-based diets to a calorie-restricted traditional diet for weight loss. Nutrition, 46, 7-13.
2. Dinu, M., Abbate, R., Gensini, G. F., Casini, A., & Sofi, F. (2017). Vegetarian, vegan diets and multiple health outcomes: A systematic review with meta-analysis of observational studies. Critical Reviews in Food Science and Nutrition, 57(17), 3640-3649.
3. Wright, N., Wilson, L., Smith, M., Duncan, B., & McHugh, P. (2017). The BROAD study: A randomized controlled trial using a whole food plant-based diet in the community for obesity, ischaemic heart disease, or diabetes. Nutrition & Diabetes, 7(3), e256.
4. Barnard, N. D., Levin, S. M., & Yokoyama, Y. (2015). A systematic review and meta-analysis of changes in body weight in clinical trials of vegetarian diets. Journal of the Academy of Nutrition and Dietetics, 115(6), 954-969.
5. Satija, A., Bhupathiraju, S. N., Spiegelman, D., Chiuve, S. E., Manson, J. E., Willett, W., ... & Hu, F. B. (2017). Healthful and unhealthful plant-based diets and the risk of coronary heart disease in US adults. Journal of the American College of Cardiology, 70(4), 411-422.
6. Tuso, P. J., Ismail, M. H., Ha, B. P., & Bartolotto, C. (2013). Nutritional update for physicians: plant-based diets. The Permanente Journal, 17(2), 61-66.

Food as Medicine: Harnessing the Healing Power of Diet

Food has been an integral part of human existence since time immemorial, serving as a source of sustenance, pleasure, and cultural identity. Beyond its role in satisfying hunger and pleasing the palate, however, food possesses incredible therapeutic potential.

This reinforces the concept that nutrition is not just about sustenance; it is also a form of medicine that can prevent, mitigate, and even reverse disease.

In this section, we explore the concept of food as medicine, unveiling the healing potential of a high raw plant-based diet in addressing specific health concerns as we delve into the remarkable healing power of a high raw plant-based diet.

The Age-Old Wisdom of Food as Medicine

The famous quote "Let food be thy medicine and medicine be thy food" is often attributed to Hippocrates, the Greek physician who is widely considered the Father of Medicine. While this quote cannot be found in any of Hippocrates' writings, it started to emerge around 1926 and gained popularity in the 1970s. Although the quote cannot be confirmed as coming from Hippocrates himself, it does reflect his emphasis on the importance of nutrition and dietary measures in maintaining good health.

In fact, dietary measures play a central role in the original Hippocratic Oath that emphasized the application of dietetic and lifestyle measures to help the sick to the best of a doctor's ability and judgment. This section of the Oath highlights the importance of protecting patients from harm and injustice through these measures as follows: "I will apply dietetic and lifestyle measures to help the sick to my best ability and judgment; I will protect them from harm and injustice".

Hippocrates clearly believed that food could serve as both excellent medicine and bad medicine, depending on its quality and suitability for an individual's condition. His writings also suggest that certain foods can have curative effects, while others may exacerbate illness. His ancient medical perspective also acknowledges that the impact of food on health can vary from case to case, stating: "In food excellent medicine can be found, in food bad medicine can be found; good and bad are relative".

Although Hippocrates did not explicitly equate food with medicine, his remarkable emphasis on dietetic measures underscores the significance he believed they play in maintaining good health.

Furthermore, his holistic approach to medicine encompassed not only dietary interventions but also exercise, with walking being a particularly recommended form of physical activity. He stated as follows "Walking is a natural exercise, more than any other form of physical exercise".

While Hippocrates' exact words may not have included the famous quote, his wise teachings have laid the foundation for understanding the vital role of nutrition in overall well-being.

The notion of food as medicine was not a novel concept unique to Hippocrates, however. Other ancient cultural healing modalities, such as Ayurveda in India and Traditional Chinese Medicine, have recognized the profound impact of diet on health for thousands of years. These traditions viewed food not only as a means of nourishment but also as a tool for preventing and treating ailments.

In recent times, modern medicine has begun to rekindle its relationship with food as a therapeutic agent. Researchers and healthcare professionals are increasingly recognizing that the foods we consume can either contribute to or mitigate various health conditions. A high raw plant-based diet is at the forefront of this dietary revolution, offering an abundance of healing potential.

The Healing Power of a High Raw Plant-Based Diet

As we have now established, a high raw plant-based diet, rooted in whole, unprocessed plant foods, is a nutritional powerhouse with the potential to prevent and alleviate a wide range of health issues. Let's explore further how this dietary approach harnesses the healing power of food:

- **Anti-Inflammatory Properties:** Chronic inflammation is at the core of many chronic diseases, including heart disease, diabetes, and autoimmune conditions. A high raw plant-based diet is inherently anti-inflammatory, thanks to its rich content of antioxidants, phytonutrients, and omega-3 fatty acids. These compounds combat inflammation at the cellular level, reducing the risk of disease and promoting healing.

- **Cardiovascular Health:** Heart disease remains a leading cause of death globally. A plant-based diet, especially one with a raw emphasis, can significantly reduce the risk of heart disease. It lowers cholesterol levels, normalizes blood pressure, supports healthy blood vessels, and enhances overall cardiovascular function.

- **Diabetes Management:** Type 2 diabetes is often related to lifestyle factors, including diet. Plant-based diets, particularly those high in raw foods, have been shown to improve insulin sensitivity, regulate blood sugar levels, and reduce the need for diabetes medications. This dietary approach empowers individuals to manage and even reverse their diabetes.

- **Weight Management:** Maintaining a healthy weight is a critical aspect of overall health. A high raw plant-based diet supports weight management by providing nutrient-dense, low-calorie foods that promote satiety and reduce overeating. It is an effective strategy for achieving and maintaining a healthy weight.

- **Cancer Prevention:** The phytonutrients found abundantly in raw plant foods have potent anti-cancer properties. These compounds help neutralize carcinogens, inhibit the growth of cancer cells, and support DNA repair mechanisms. While not a standalone treatment, a plant-based diet can play a role in cancer prevention and adjunctive therapy.

- **Digestive Health:** A diet rich in raw plant foods is gentle on the digestive system. The fiber and enzymes in these foods support regular bowel movements, prevent constipation, and promote a balanced gut microbiota. This contributes to overall digestive wellness.

- **Mental Health:** Emerging research suggests a link between diet and mental health. A high raw plant-based diet is associated with a reduced risk of depression and anxiety. The nutrient-dense nature of this diet supports brain health and the production of neurotransmitters that influence mood.

- **Immune Support:** The immune system relies on proper nutrition to function optimally. A high raw plant-based diet provides the essential vitamins, minerals, and antioxidants required for immune defense, reducing the risk of infections and supporting immune-mediated healing.

- **Bone Health:** Contrary to common misconceptions, a well-planned high raw plant-based diet can support bone health. Plant foods like leafy greens taken along with a source of Vitamin C, as well as almonds, and fortified plant-based milk provide calcium, while the magnesium and vitamin K2 these foods provide are essential for bone metabolism.

- **Longevity and Vitality:** A high raw plant-based diet is associated with enhanced longevity and vitality. It promotes healthy aging by reducing the risk of chronic diseases, supporting cognitive function, and preserving physical mobility.

Practical Tips for Harnessing Food as Medicine

If you want to enjoy the benefits of harnessing food as your medicine to maintain or improve your overall health and wellness, then you can incorporate the following tips into your dietary plan.

1. **Embrace Variety:** Incorporate a wide range of raw plant foods into your diet, including fruits, vegetables, leafy greens, nuts, seeds, and legumes. Diversity ensures you receive a broad spectrum of nutrients.

2. **Focus on Whole Foods:** Choose whole, unprocessed foods whenever possible. These foods retain their natural goodness and are free from additives and preservatives.

3. **Mindful Eating:** Practice mindful eating by savoring each bite, chewing food thoroughly, and paying attention to hunger and fullness cues.

4. **Hydration:** Stay well-hydrated by drinking plenty of water and herbal teas. Hydration is essential for overall health and healing.

5. **Balanced Macronutrients:** Strive for a balanced intake of macronutrients, including carbohydrates, healthy fats, and plant-based proteins.

6. **Consult a Healthcare Professional:** If you have specific health concerns or conditions, consult with a healthcare professional or registered dietitian to develop a personalized dietary plan.

Food as Your Ally in Health Maintenance

Overall, incorporating a high raw plant-based diet into your lifestyle is a powerful step toward harnessing the healing power of food. While this dietary approach is not a panacea, it can be a potent ally in preventing, managing, and even reversing various health conditions.

By embracing the age-old wisdom of food as medicine and nourishing your body with the vitality of raw plant foods, you can embark on a journey of holistic healing and well-being.

Section References:

1. Tuso, P. J., Ismail, M. H., Ha, B. P., & Bartolotto, C. (2013). Nutritional update for physicians: plant-based diets. The Permanente Journal, 17(2), 61-66.
2. Satija, A., Bhupathiraju, S. N., Rimm, E. B., Spiegelman, D., Chiuve, S. E., Borgi, L., ... & Hu, F. B. (2016). Plant-based dietary patterns and incidence of type 2 diabetes in US men and women: results from three prospective cohort studies. PLoS Medicine, 13(6), e1002039.
3. Tonstad, S., Stewart, K., Oda, K., Batech, M., & Herring, R. P. (2013). Vegetarian diets and incidence of diabetes in the Adventist Health Study-2. Nutrition, Metabolism and Cardiovascular Diseases, 23(4), 292-299.
4. Dinu, M., Abbate, R., Gensini, G. F., Casini, A., & Sofi, F. (2017). Vegetarian, vegan diets and multiple health outcomes: a systematic review with meta-analysis of observational studies. Critical Reviews in Food Science and Nutrition, 57(17), 3640-3649.
5. Micha, R., Peñalvo, J. L., Cudhea, F., Imamura, F., Rehm, C. D., & Mozaffarian, D. (2017). Association Between Dietary Factors and Mortality From Heart Disease, Stroke, and Type 2 Diabetes. JAMA, 317(9), 912–924.
6. Li, D. (2013). Effect of the vegetarian diet on non-communicable diseases. Journal of the Science of Food and Agriculture, 93(12), 2999-3005.
7. Olfert, M. D., Wattick, R. A., & Hagedorn, R. L. (2018). A vegetarian diet may be associated with a lower risk of metabolic syndrome and metabolic syndrome components in rural Southwestern Oklahoma adults. The Journal of Nutrition, Health & Aging, 22(6), 710-716.
8. Turner-McGrievy, G. M., & Wirth, M. D. (2017). Comparison of plant-based diets to a calorie-restricted traditional diet for weight loss. Nutrition, 46, 7-13.
9. Satija, A., Bhupathiraju, S. N., Spiegelman, D., Chiuve, S. E., Manson, J. E., Willett, W., ... & Hu, F. B. (2017). Healthful and unhealthful plant-based diets and the risk of coronary heart disease in US adults. Journal of the American College of Cardiology, 70(4), 411-422.
10. Kim, H., Caulfield, L. E., Garcia-Larsen, V., Steffen, L. M., Coresh, J., & Rebholz, C. M. (2019). Plant-based diets are associated with a lower

risk of incident cardiovascular disease, cardiovascular disease mortality, and all-cause mortality in a general population of middle-aged adults. Journal of the American Heart Association, 8(16), e012865.

Therapeutic Diets: Tailoring Nutrition for Specific Conditions

Certain health conditions require specialized dietary approaches for optimal management and healing. We delve into therapeutic diets that are rooted in the principles of a high raw plant-based diet, showcasing their potential in addressing conditions such as diabetes, autoimmune diseases, and cancer.

Explore the science behind therapeutic diets, including the low-glycemic index diet for diabetes management and the anti-inflammatory diet for autoimmune conditions. Discover how a high raw plant-based diet can provide the foundation for these therapeutic approaches, offering hope and healing for those facing specific health challenges.

As we navigate the terrain of healing through food, keep in mind that the principles of a high raw plant-based diet remain at the forefront of our exploration. The vibrant, nutrient-rich foods found in nature are our allies in promoting wellness, preventing disease, and harnessing the remarkable power of nutrition.

Through these sections, you will gain insights into the intricate relationship between nutrition and health, unlocking the potential of a high raw plant-based diet to transform your well-being. It is my hope that this knowledge empowers you to make informed choices and embark on a journey of healing and vitality.

Despite its use as a healing modality, remember that nutrition is not a one-size-fits-all concept. It's a dynamic and adaptable aspect of our lives, capable of addressing specific health concerns and conditions. Therapeutic diets are specialized dietary approaches designed to support the management and treatment of various health issues.

In this section, we'll explore the potential of therapeutic diets, with a strong emphasis on the healing capacity of a high raw plant-based diet for specific conditions. Let us now embark on this transformative journey through the healing power of nutrition, where food becomes not just sustenance but a source of profound well-being and vitality.

The Art of Therapeutic Diets

Therapeutic diets have been used for centuries to address health challenges and enhance well-being. They are rooted in the understanding that the foods we consume can be powerful allies in our journey to health.

Despite their widely-acknowledged and science-based benefits, therapeutic diets are not a replacement for medical treatment but a complementary approach that can significantly impact the management and even the reversal of certain conditions.

A High Raw Plant-Based Diet as a Therapeutic Approach

A high raw plant-based diet, characterized by the consumption of a significant portion of raw, uncooked plant foods focusing on fruits and leafy greens, offers a remarkable platform for therapeutic nutrition. This ancestral and physiologically-appropriate dietary approach is versatile, nutrient-dense, and abundant in health-promoting compounds.

When it comes to using it as a therapeutic approach, let's explore how a high raw plant-based diet can be tailored to address several specific conditions in the following sections. Keep in mind that this is not an exhaustive list of health conditions that can be substantially improved by following this natural and healthful diet, but instead just a few for which this diet has been firmly established to have therapeutic benefits.

Heart Disease

Condition: Heart disease, including conditions like atherosclerosis and hypertension, is a leading cause of death worldwide.

Therapeutic Diet: A high raw plant-based diet is inherently heart-healthy. It supports cardiovascular health by reducing cholesterol levels, normalizing blood pressure, and enhancing the function of blood vessels. Foods rich in antioxidants, such as berries and leafy greens, help combat oxidative stress, while the diet's low saturated fat content minimizes plaque buildup in arteries.

Diabetes

Condition: Diabetes, especially type 2 diabetes, is often linked to lifestyle factors, obesity and diet.

Therapeutic Diet: A high raw plant-based diet can help regulate blood sugar levels and improve insulin sensitivity. It emphasizes low-glycemic foods, such as fruits, leafy greens, whole grains, legumes, and non-starchy vegetables, to prevent spikes in blood sugar. The fiber-rich nature of the diet also contributes to blood sugar control.

Digestive Disorders

Condition: Digestive disorders like irritable bowel syndrome (IBS) and inflammatory bowel disease (IBD) can be characterized by symptoms such as abdominal pain, bloating, and irregular bowel movements.

Therapeutic Diet: A high raw plant-based diet, when well-tolerated, can provide relief for some individuals with digestive disorders. It is gentle on the digestive system and rich in fiber, which can alleviate symptoms of IBS. Additionally, certain raw plant foods, like aloe vera and ginger, have soothing properties for the gut.

Cancer Prevention and Treatment

Condition: Cancer is a complex group of diseases with various risk factors, including diet.

Therapeutic Diet: A high raw plant-based diet is associated with a reduced risk of certain cancers. The phytonutrients and antioxidants in raw plant foods help neutralize carcinogens and inhibit the growth of cancer cells. While not a guarantee against cancer, this diet can contribute to prevention.

Weight Management

Condition: Excess body weight is linked to a range of health issues, including heart disease, diabetes, and joint problems.

Therapeutic Diet: A high raw plant-based diet is naturally supportive of weight management. Its low caloric density makes it easier to control calorie intake, and the fiber content promotes satiety, reducing overeating. This dietary approach empowers individuals to achieve and maintain a healthy weight.

Autoimmune Diseases

Condition: Autoimmune diseases occur when the immune system mistakenly attacks the body's own tissues, leading to chronic inflammation and various symptoms.

Therapeutic Diet: While dietary strategies for autoimmune diseases can be complex and individualized, a high raw plant-based diet can serve as a foundation. Its anti-inflammatory nature may help mitigate symptoms, and the abundance of antioxidants can support immune function and reduce inflammation.

Mental Health

Condition: Emerging research suggests a connection between diet and mental health, with certain dietary patterns influencing mood and well-being.

Therapeutic Diet: A high raw plant-based diet, rich in nutrients that support brain health, may have a positive impact on mental well-being. It provides essential vitamins, minerals, and antioxidants that play a role in neurotransmitter production and mood regulation.

Kidney Health

Condition: Chronic kidney disease (CKD) requires dietary modifications to manage electrolyte imbalances and reduce the strain on the kidneys.

Therapeutic Diet: A high raw plant-based diet can be adapted for individuals with CKD by limiting high-potassium and high-phosphorus foods while emphasizing kidney-friendly options. Careful planning and consultation with a healthcare provider or registered dietitian are essential.

Practical Considerations for Therapeutic Diets

If you want to enjoy the benefits of harnessing food as a therapeutic way to maintain or improve your overall health and wellness, then you can incorporate the following tips into your dietary plan.

1. **Individualization:** Therapeutic diets should be tailored to the individual's specific condition, preferences, and dietary tolerances. Consulting with a healthcare provider or registered dietitian is crucial for personalized guidance.

2. **Monitoring:** Regular monitoring of health markers, such as blood sugar levels or cholesterol levels, is important when following a therapeutic diet. Adjustments may be needed as health improves.
3. **Supplementation:** Depending on the specific condition and dietary restrictions, supplementation with certain nutrients may be necessary. Consult with a healthcare provider for guidance on supplements.
4. **Patient Education:** Individuals following therapeutic diets should receive proper education on meal planning, food choices, and cooking techniques to ensure success.
5. **Lifestyle Factors:** Therapeutic diets are most effective when combined with other healthy lifestyle practices, such as regular physical activity and stress management.

The Therapeutic Healing Potential of a High Raw Plant-Based Diet

Therapeutic diets have the potential to transform health and well-being. A high raw plant-based diet, with its focus on whole, unprocessed, nutrient-dense foods, offers a versatile and powerful approach to addressing specific health conditions.

Whether you're seeking to prevent chronic diseases, manage or even reverse existing conditions, or optimize your overall well-being, the healing potential of food as medicine is a path worth exploring.

Section References:

1. Tuso, P. J., Ismail, M. H., Ha, B. P., & Bartolotto, C. (2013). Nutritional update for physicians: plant-based diets. The Permanente Journal, 17(2), 61-66.
2. Satija, A., Bhupathiraju, S. N., Rimm, E. B., Spiegelman, D., Chiuve, S. E., Borgi, L., ... & Hu, F. B. (2016). Plant-based dietary patterns and incidence of type 2 diabetes in US men and women: results from three prospective cohort studies. PLoS Medicine, 13(6), e1002039.
3. Dinu, M., Abbate, R., Gensini, G. F., Casini, A., & Sofi, F. (2017). Vegetarian, vegan diets and multiple health outcomes: a systematic review with meta-analysis of observational studies. Critical Reviews in Food Science and Nutrition, 57(17), 3640-3649.
4. Turner-McGrievy, G. M., & Wirth, M. D. (2017). Comparison of plant-based diets to a calorie-restricted traditional diet for weight loss. Nutrition, 46, 7-13.
5. Satija, A., Bhupathiraju, S. N., Spiegelman, D., Chiuve, S. E., Manson, J. E., Willett, W., ... & Hu, F. B. (2017). Healthful and unhealthful plant-

based diets and the risk of coronary heart disease in US adults. Journal of the American College of Cardiology, 70(4), 411-422.

6. Kim, H., Caulfield, L. E., Garcia-Larsen, V., Steffen, L. M., Coresh, J., & Rebholz, C. M. (2019). Plant-based diets are associated with a lower risk of incident cardiovascular disease, cardiovascular disease mortality, and all-cause mortality in a general population of middle-aged adults. Journal of the American Heart Association, 8(16), e012865.

7. Barnard, N. D., Levin, S. M., & Yokoyama, Y. (2015). A systematic review and meta-analysis of changes in body weight in clinical trials of vegetarian diets. Journal of the Academy of Nutrition and Dietetics, 115(6), 954-969.

Chapter References:

1. Mozaffarian, D., Benjamin, E. J., Go, A. S., Arnett, D. K., Blaha, M. J., Cushman, M., ... & Turner, M. B. (2016). Heart disease and stroke statistics—2016 update: a report from the American Heart Association. Circulation, 133(4), e38-e360.

2. Guarner, F., & Malagelada, J. R. (2003). Gut flora in health and disease. The Lancet, 361(9356), 512-519.

3. Gómez-Pinilla, F. (2008). Brain foods: the effects of nutrients on brain function. Nature Reviews Neuroscience, 9(7), 568-578.

4. Calder, P. C., Carr, A. C., Gombart, A. F., & Eggersdorfer, M. (2020). Optimal nutritional status for a well-functioning immune system is an important factor to protect against viral infections. Nutrients, 12(4), 1181.

5. Franz, M. J., Boucher, J. L., Evert, A. B., MacLeod, J., & Academy of Nutrition and Dietetics. (2014). Evidence-based diabetes nutrition therapy recommendations are effective: the key is individualization. Diabetes, Metabolic Syndrome and Obesity: Targets and Therapy, 7, 65-72.

6. Barnard, N. D., Nicholson, A., & Howard, J. L. (1995). The medical costs attributable to meat consumption. Preventive Medicine, 24(6), 646-655.

64

PART III: MAKING BETTER FOOD CHOICES

THE ART OF MINDFUL EATING

In our fast-paced world, the act of eating has often become a rushed and mindless activity. We eat on the go, in front of screens, or while multitasking, disconnected from the experience of nourishing our bodies.

This disconnect can lead to overeating, poor food choices, and an inability to truly savor and appreciate the flavors and textures of our meals. Mindful eating is a practice that seeks to change this by bringing awareness and consciousness to our eating habits.

When combined with a high raw plant-based diet, mindful eating becomes a powerful tool for improving both physical and mental well-being.

What is Mindful Eating?

At its core, mindful eating is about paying full attention to the act of eating in the present moment, without judgment. It involves using all of your senses to truly experience your food—sight, smell, taste, touch, and even sound.

Mindful eating encourages you to slow down, savor each bite, and make deliberate choices about what and how much you eat.

The Benefits of Mindful Eating

Mindful eating offers a multitude of benefits for both physical and psychological health. Here are some of the key advantages:

- **Weight Management:** One of the most well-documented benefits of mindful eating is its effectiveness in weight management. By becoming more attuned to hunger and fullness cues, individuals are less likely to overeat and are better equipped to maintain a healthy weight.

- **Improved Digestion:** Mindful eating encourages thorough chewing and proper digestion. This can reduce digestive discomfort and promote better nutrient absorption.
- **Enhanced Food Appreciation:** When you truly savor each bite, you gain a greater appreciation for the flavors and textures of your food. This can lead to increased satisfaction with your meals, even if they are simple and comprised of raw plant foods.
- **Better Food Choices:** Mindful eating helps you become more aware of the types of foods you consume. It can lead to a greater inclination toward choosing whole, nutrient-dense foods like fruits, vegetables, nuts, and seeds.
- **Emotional Eating Awareness:** Mindful eating can help individuals recognize emotional triggers for overeating or unhealthy food choices. This awareness allows for more constructive responses to emotional needs.
- **Reduced Stress:** The practice of mindfulness, including mindful eating, has been shown to reduce stress levels. Lower stress can have a positive impact on overall health.
- **Improved Relationship with Food:** Mindful eating fosters a healthier and more positive relationship with food. It can help break the cycle of restrictive diets and disordered eating patterns.

How to Practice Mindful Eating

Mindful eating is a practice that can be cultivated over time. Here are some practical steps to get you started as a mindful eater:

1. **Create a Calm Environment:** Find a quiet and peaceful space to eat your meals. Turn off distractions like the TV or computer, and put away your phone.
2. **Engage Your Senses:** Before taking your first bite, take a moment to observe your food. Notice its colors, textures, and shapes. Inhale deeply to appreciate the aroma.
3. **Eat Slowly:** Chew each bite thoroughly and savor the flavors. Put your utensils down between bites to pace yourself.
4. **Tune into Hunger and Fullness:** Pay attention to your body's hunger and fullness signals. Eat when you're moderately hungry and stop when you're satisfied, not overly full.
5. **Practice Gratitude:** Take a moment to express gratitude for your food and the nourishment it provides.
6. **Mindful Portion Control:** Be mindful of portion sizes,

especially when it comes to calorie-dense foods. Raw plant-based foods tend to be less calorie-dense than processed or animal-based foods, but portion control remains important.

7. **Listen to Your Body:** Your body knows what it needs. If you find yourself craving a particular food, it may be because your body is signaling a specific nutritional need. Listen to these cues.

8. **Be Nonjudgmental:** Avoid self-criticism or judgment during your mindful eating practice. If you notice yourself making negative judgments about your food choices or eating habits, simply acknowledge them and let them go.

Mindful Eating and a High Raw Plant-Based Diet

Mindful eating and a high raw plant-based diet are a natural fit. The simplicity and freshness of raw plant foods make them ideal for savoring and appreciating each bite. Here's some of the ways in which they complement each other:

- **Sensory Richness:** Raw plant foods offer a sensory-rich eating experience. The vibrant colors, crisp textures, and diverse flavors of fruits, vegetables, and nuts can be truly savored in a mindful eating practice.

- **Natural Satisfaction:** A high raw plant-based diet prioritizes nutrient-dense foods, which can lead to increased satisfaction with meals. You'll feel more content with your choices and less likely to overeat.

- **Whole Foods Emphasis:** Mindful eating encourages choosing whole, unprocessed foods. This aligns perfectly with the principles of a high raw plant-based diet, which emphasizes minimally processed, whole foods.

- **Emotional Eating Awareness:** A high raw plant-based diet combined with mindful eating can help individuals recognize and address emotional eating patterns, fostering a healthier relationship with food.

- **Mindful Meal Preparation:** The process of preparing raw plant-based meals can itself be a mindful practice. Engaging with the colors and textures of fresh produce can be a form of meditation.

Incorporating Mindful Eating into Your Routine

Like any skill, mindful eating takes practice. Start by setting aside at least one meal per day to eat mindfully. As you become more comfortable with the practice, you can gradually extend it to more meals and snacks.

Remember that mindfulness is not an all-or-nothing endeavor. Even moments of mindful eating can have a positive impact on your relationship with food and your overall well-being.

The key is to approach each meal with intention and presence, savoring the simple pleasures of nourishing your body with high-quality, raw plant-based foods.

Section References:

1. Kristeller, J. L., & Wolever, R. Q. (2011). Mindfulness-Based Eating Awareness Training for Treating Binge Eating Disorder: The Conceptual Foundation. Eating Disorders, 19(1), 49-61.
2. Daubenmier, J., Kristeller, J., Hecht, F. M., Maninger, N., Kuwata, M., Jhaveri, K., ... & Epel, E. (2011). Mindfulness Intervention for Stress Eating to Reduce Cortisol and Abdominal Fat among Overweight and Obese Women: An Exploratory Randomized Controlled Study. Journal of Obesity, 2011, 651936.
3. Mantzios, M., & Wilson, J. C. (2015). Exploring Mindfulness and Mindful Eating as Supportive of Weight Management. Psychology & Health, 30(2), 165-173.
4. O'Reilly, G. A., Cook, L., Spruijt-Metz, D., & Black, D. S. (2014). Mindfulness-based interventions for obesity-related eating behaviours: a literature review. Obesity Reviews, 15(6), 453-461.
5. Albers, S. (2003). Eating Mindfully: How to End Mindless Eating and Enjoy a Balanced Relationship with Food. New Harbinger Publications.

GROCERY SHOPPING FOR HEALTH

One of the most powerful ways to transition to a high raw plant-based diet is by being mindful of your grocery shopping habits. The choices you make at the grocery store can set the foundation for your nutritional healing journey.

By primarily shopping in the produce and bulk bin section of your local grocery store, you can largely limit your food consumption to raw plant foods, fostering better health and vitality as has previously been discussed in this book.

The Produce Section: Your Nutrient Goldmine

When you enter a grocery store, the produce section should become your first destination. This vibrant and colorful area is a treasure trove of raw plant-based foods that can nourish your body in countless ways. Here's what you'll most likely find there:

- **A Rainbow of Fresh Fruits and Vegetables:** The produce section is a visual feast of fruits and vegetables in a wide range of colors. Each color represents different phytonutrients, vitamins, and minerals essential for optimal health. For instance, red and orange fruits like tomatoes and bell peppers are rich in vitamin C and antioxidants, while leafy greens like kale and spinach provide an abundance of vitamin A and Swiss chard is especially rich in vitamin K.

- **Seasonal Variety:** Shopping for seasonal produce not only ensures freshness but also supports local agriculture and reduces your carbon footprint. Plus, seasonal fruits and vegetables are often at their peak in terms of flavor and nutrition.

- **Organic Options:** Whenever possible, opt for organic produce, especially for items listed on the Environmental Working Group's "Dirty Dozen" list, which includes fruits and vegetables that tend to have higher pesticide residues when conventionally grown. Organic choices can reduce your exposure to harmful chemicals.

- **Fresh Herbs and Spices:** Don't forget to explore the fresh herbs and spices available. These add flavor and depth to your raw plant-based meals without the need for excess salt or processed seasonings. You can use fresh basil and garlic to make a delicious pesto sauce for raw crackers and spiralized veggies.

The Bulk Bin Section: Whole, Unprocessed Staples

The bulk bin section is your gateway to whole, unprocessed staples that are essential for a high raw plant-based diet. Here, you can find a variety of raw nuts, seeds, dried fruits, and whole grains.

Raw nuts and seeds are essential components of a high raw plant-based diet and provide valuable fats and calories for those looking to maintain their ideal weight. Look for them in the bulk bin section to ensure they are in their natural, unprocessed state.

However, it's important to note that not all items in the bulk bin section are raw, even if they appear uncooked. Almonds, cashews, and oats, for example, are often pasteurized or heat-treated, so it's essential to seek out explicitly labeled "raw" options if you want to maintain a strict raw diet for its health benefits.

Canned, Bottled, and Packaged Foods: Proceed with Caution

In your pursuit of a high raw plant-based diet, it's advisable to steer clear of canned, bottled, and packaged foods that do not explicitly have "raw" on the label.

Even some fermented foods with live cultures may have been cooked before fermentation was started. If you want to eat fermented foods, you can often use the live cultures obtained from commercial foods to seed a fermentation process you perform at home. This can work with popular fermented foods and drinks like kombucha, sauerkraut, plant-based yogurts and kefirs, and kim chi. If you wish to create fermented foods, make sure you research how to do so safely.

Another issue you may come across when shopping for raw foods is that many processed foods are heated during preparation, which can destroy essential nutrients and enzymes present in raw plant-based foods. Additionally, these products may contain additives, preservatives, salt, and hidden sugars that are not aligned with the principles of a high raw diet.

Navigating the Aisles for Raw Options

While the produce and bulk bin sections will be your primary destinations, you may still need to explore other parts of the grocery store for specific raw ingredients or pantry staples. Here's some tips on how to navigate the aisles for raw plant-based grocery items you may wish to buy:

- **Condiments and Dressings:** Opt for raw condiments and dressings that use fresh herbs, fruits, and vegetables as their base. You can also make your own raw salad dressings at home using ingredients like olive oil, vinegar, lemon juice, and spices.

- **Plant-Based Milks:** Look for unsweetened, unfortified and raw plant-based milks like almond milk or coconut milk. While some brands offer raw versions that are simply made from blended nuts and water, although these are rare. In general, you will probably just want to buy raw nuts, grains and/or seeds and make plant-based milks yourself by using a blender to combine them with high quality water or raw coconut milk.

- **Dried Fruits, Nuts and Seeds:** When selecting dried fruits, check for options that do not contain added sugars, preservatives, or sulfur dioxide. Additionally, choose only raw nuts and seeds for snacking since those that have been roasted, steamed or pasteurized are not raw.

- **Whole Grains:** If you choose to include grains in your diet, opt for raw, sprouted grains like quinoa, spelt, buckwheat, oat groats, and wheat berries. These grains are minimally processed and retain more of their natural nutrients that are boosted by the sprouting process.

- **Freshly Pressed Juices:** Some grocery stores offer freshly pressed juices made from raw fruits and vegetables. These can be a convenient way to incorporate raw nutrients into your diet, but tread carefully here since juices are generally best made at home from fresh produce to assure that they are raw and have the highest nutritional benefits.

- **Specialty Aisles:** In health food or specialty sections of the store, you may find packaged raw food items like kale chips or raw energy bars. However, be cautious and check ingredient labels for any additives, sugar, salt or processed components.

Online Shopping for Raw Ingredients

In addition to physical grocery stores, consider exploring online options for sourcing raw ingredients. Many online retailers offer a wide range of raw nuts, seeds, dried fruits, and specialty items that can be challenging to find locally.

When shopping online, carefully read product descriptions to ensure items are labeled as raw and minimally processed. Thankfully, Amazon.com has an especially wide range of raw foods due to its association with Whole Foods.

Shopping for Produce at Farmer's Markets

Local farmer's markets offer a delightful alternative to traditional grocery stores when you're seeking fresh, locally sourced, and often organic produce for your high raw plant-based diet. Here's how to make the most of your farmer's market shopping experience:

- **Seasonal Bounty:** Farmer's markets excel in offering seasonal produce at its peak of flavor and nutritional value. By shopping seasonally, you not only enjoy a variety of fresh foods but also support local agriculture.
- **Organic Options:** Many small-scale farmers at these markets prioritize organic and sustainable farming practices. While not all vendors may be certified organic, they often employ eco-friendly methods that prioritize soil health and reduce chemical use.
- **Freshness Guaranteed:** The produce you find at farmer's markets has often been harvested recently, ensuring optimal freshness and nutrient retention. This is particularly advantageous for raw plant-based enthusiasts seeking the highest nutritional value.
- **Unique Finds:** Farmer's markets often feature unique and heirloom varieties of fruits and vegetables that you may not encounter in conventional grocery stores. These specialty items can add excitement and diversity to your high raw diet.
- **Build Relationships:** Building a rapport with local farmers can be rewarding. They can provide insights into the foods they grow, share preparation tips, and even accommodate special requests if

you're looking for specific raw items.

- **Supporting Local Agriculture:** Shopping at farmer's markets directly supports local farmers and the community's economy. Your purchases contribute to sustainable agriculture and reduce the carbon footprint associated with food transportation.

Overall, shopping at farmer's markets provides an opportunity to connect directly with local farmers and artisans, fostering a sense of community and sustainability while ensuring the highest freshness and quality of your food.

Subscribing to Produce Boxes from a Farming Collective

Another excellent option for sourcing fresh, raw plant-based ingredients is by subscribing to produce boxes from a farming collective or community-supported agriculture (CSA) program.

These programs allow you to receive regular deliveries of seasonal and locally grown produce directly from the farm. Here's why this approach aligns perfectly with your high raw plant-based diet:

- **Farm-Fresh Deliveries:** Subscribing to a CSA or farming collective means you'll receive a regular supply of farm-fresh produce. These deliveries often include a variety of fruits, vegetables, and sometimes herbs, ensuring a diverse and nutritious raw diet.
- **Seasonal Variety:** Like farmer's markets, CSA programs provide seasonal produce, which is at its nutritional peak and abundant in flavors. You'll be inspired to create raw culinary masterpieces with the ever-changing selection.
- **Supporting Local Farmers:** By participating in a CSA or farming collective, you directly support local farmers and sustainable agriculture. Your subscription fees contribute to the livelihoods of these farmers, fostering a sense of community and environmental responsibility.
- **Reduced Food Miles:** CSA programs emphasize local sourcing, which means your food travels fewer miles from farm to table. This reduces the carbon footprint associated with long-distance transportation, aligning with sustainability goals.
- **Connection to the Source:** Subscribers often have opportunities to visit the farm, attend workshops, or engage in community events. This connection to the source of your food enhances your appreciation for raw plant-based nutrition.

- **Farm-to-Table Experience:** CSA programs offer a unique farm-to-table experience. You'll have a deeper understanding of where your food comes from and how it's grown, reinforcing your commitment to a high raw diet.
- **Customizable Options:** Some CSA programs allow subscribers to customize their boxes or add specific items, ensuring you receive the raw ingredients that align with your dietary preferences.

Building Your Raw Plant-Based Pantry from Diverse Sources

Grocery shopping for a high raw plant-based diet is an exciting journey toward better health and vitality. By focusing on the produce and bulk bin sections of your local store and selecting raw options thoughtfully in other sections of the store or online, you can fill your pantry with whole, unprocessed staples.

This approach not only supports your nutritional healing but also aligns with the principles of a diet that emphasizes the consumption of raw plant foods.

Furthermore, shopping for raw plant-based foods can be an enriching experience when you explore diverse avenues like farmer's markets and CSA subscriptions. These excellent options not only provide you with access to the freshest and most nutritious produce but also allow you to actively support local agriculture and sustainable farming practices.

Whether you choose the vibrant atmosphere of a farmer's market or the convenience of regular produce box deliveries, both approaches align perfectly with the principles of a high raw plant-based diet, emphasizing fresh, whole, and minimally processed foods.

Remember to read labels carefully, choose organic options when possible, and stay mindful of sourcing truly raw ingredients, especially for nuts, seeds, and grains. With patience and a commitment to mindful grocery and produce farm shopping, you'll be well on your way to reaping the abundant health benefits of a high raw plant-based diet.

Section References:

1. Berrin, S., & Johnson, E. J. (2015). The Storied History of the Food Guide Pyramid. Nutrition Today, 50(6), 282-292.
2. Bode, A. M., & Dong, Z. (2015). The Amazing and Mighty Ginger. In Benzie I. F. F. and Wachtel-Galor S. (Eds.), Herbal Medicine: Biomolecular and Clinical Aspects. CRC Press/Taylor & Francis.

3. Jia, Z., Tang, M., Wu, J., Ni, Y., Zhang, X., & Duan, J. (2016). The influence of ripening stages on the levels of phenolics, isothiocyanates, carotenoids, and antioxidant activity of goji berry (Lycium barbarum L.). Food Chemistry, 209, 26-34.

4. Escribano, J., Pedreño, M. A., García-Carmona, F., & Muñoz, R. (1998). Characterization of the enzyme(s) responsible for the de-astringency phenomenon induced by carbon dioxide in persimmon. Journal of Agricultural and Food Chemistry, 46(11), 4571-4577.

5. Stuetz, W., Prapaveessai, T., & Popluechai, S. (2010). Comparison of nutrient content

6. United States Department of Agriculture. (2019). Benefits of Buying Fresh, Local Produce. Retrieved from:
https://www.fns.usda.gov/farmers-markets/benefits-buying-fresh-locally-grown-produce

7. Hardesty, S. (2014). What Do We Know about the Affordability of Local Food? A Review of Literature on the Costs and Benefits of Purchasing from Local Producers. Retrieved from:
https://www.ams.usda.gov/sites/default/files/media/Local_Food_Short_Version.pdf

8. United States Department of Agriculture. (2018). Community Supported Agriculture. Retrieved from:
https://www.nal.usda.gov/afsic/community-supported-agriculture

PREPARING FOOD FOR WELLNESS

Transitioning to a high raw plant-based diet isn't just about selecting the right ingredients; it's also about mastering healthy raw food preparation techniques.

Understanding how to prepare raw foods creatively and safely is essential for maximizing both the nutritional value and the culinary appeal of your meals.

In this chapter, we'll explore various methods for preparing healthy and raw plant-based dishes that will not only support your well-being but also tantalize your taste buds.

Dehydration: Preserving Nutrients and Texture

Dehydration is a key technique in raw food preparation that involves removing moisture from foods while preserving their nutrients and flavors. This method is commonly used to create snacks, crackers, and fruit leathers, among other raw delights. The benefits of dehydration include:

- **Nutrient Retention:** Dehydration at low temperatures (usually below 117°F or 47.2°C that correspond to the heat of the sun on a hot day) helps preserve the vital enzymes and nutrients present in raw foods, making them available to your body.
- **Texture and Shelf Life:** Dehydrated foods maintain their original texture and can have a longer shelf life, allowing you to enjoy seasonal produce year-round.
- **Versatility:** You can dehydrate a wide range of foods, from fruits and vegetables to nuts and seeds, giving you endless possibilities for raw snacks, crackers and textured dishes.

To use a food dehydrator, simply slice or prepare your ingredients and arrange them on the dehydrator trays. Make sure to select a dehydrator with a temperature control, since you do not want to cook the food or heat it above 117 degrees.

Set the temperature to the desired level and wait for the magic to happen. Keep in mind that dehydrating times vary depending on the food and thickness, so consult your dehydrator's manual for specific guidelines.

Sun Drying: A More Natural Alternative to Dehydration

Sun drying is another method for preserving raw foods using the power of the sun. While it may not be as precise as a food dehydrator, it's a natural and energy-efficient way to create sun-dried fruits, tomatoes, and other delectable treats. Here's how it works:

- **Preparation:** Slice or halve your chosen produce, ensuring uniformity to promote even drying.
- **Drying Rack:** Place your food on a clean and dry surface, preferably a drying rack or a screen that allows air circulation.
- **Protection:** Protect the food from bugs and dust.
- **Sun Exposure:** Position the rack in direct sunlight, preferably in a location with consistent airflow. Cover the food with cheesecloth or a mesh screen to protect it from insects and debris.
- **Patience:** Sun drying can take several days, depending on the weather and humidity levels. Turn and rotate the food periodically for even drying.
- **Storage:** Once your food is thoroughly dried (it should be pliable but not moist), store it in airtight containers to maintain freshness.

Food Processing: Creating Texture and Variety

Food processing equipment can be invaluable tools for a high raw plant-based diet. These appliances can help you create diverse textures and flavors, making raw meals more interesting and satisfying. Here are some ways to use them:

- **Food Processors:** Food processors are ideal for chopping, slicing, dicing, and shredding raw ingredients. Use them to prepare salads, raw vegetable noodles, and even nut-based crusts for raw desserts.
- **Nut Butters and Sauces:** With a food processor or high-speed blender, you can make your own raw nut butters and sauces, free

from added preservatives or sugars. Just make sure that any almonds or cashews you use are fully raw and not steamed or pasteurized,

- **Seed and Nut Flours:** Grinding nuts and seeds in a food processor, strong blender or flour grinder can yield flours that serve as the base for raw crusts, bread, or desserts.

When using these appliances, ensure that your ingredients are fresh and of high quality to achieve the best results. Experiment with various textures and combinations to create raw dishes that suit your taste.

Blending: Creamy Raw Creations

Blending is a foundational technique in raw food preparation, allowing you to create smooth, creamy, and nutrient-dense concoctions. Blenders are perfect for whipping up nutrient-packed smoothies, creamy raw plant-based soups, and sauces. They break down tough fibers, making it easier for your body to absorb nutrients.

Here's how you can harness the power of blending for your high raw plant-based diet:

- **Smoothies:** Blenders are very useful for crafting vibrant, nutrient-packed smoothies. Simply combine fresh fruits, leafy greens, seeds, and liquids like water, coconut water, or plant-based milk. Blend until smooth and enjoy a wholesome meal in a glass.
- **Creamy Soups:** Raw soups are a nourishing option for a high raw diet. Blend ingredients like ripe tomatoes, cucumbers, avocados, and herbs to create chilled soups bursting with flavor.
- **Sauces and Dressings:** Blenders can effortlessly combine ingredients for raw sauces and dressings. Whisk together ingredients like olive oil, lemon juice, garlic, and fresh herbs to elevate your salads and dishes.
- **Nut and Seed Milks:** Make your own raw nut and seed milks using blenders. Soak your chosen nuts or seeds, blend with water, and strain to create dairy-free milk alternatives.

Blending is not only a convenient way to prepare raw meals but also an excellent method for breaking down cell walls and enhancing nutrient absorption.

Spiralizing: Noodles from Nature

Spiralizing is a fun and innovative technique for incorporating more raw vegetables into your diet by turning them into noodle-like strands. A spiralizer is a kitchen gadget that can transform vegetables like zucchini, carrots, and sweet potatoes into noodle shapes. Here's how to use it:

- **Selecting Vegetables:** Choose firm, fresh root vegetables and squashes for spiralizing. Common choices include zucchini, carrots, cucumbers, beets, and sweet potatoes.
- **Preparation:** Trim the ends of the vegetable and secure it in the spiralizer. Follow the manufacturer's instructions for creating noodles of your desired thickness.
- **Texture Variety:** Spiralized vegetables can be used as a base for salads, raw pasta dishes, or as a crunchy addition to wraps and bowls. They add texture and visual appeal to your raw creations.

Overall, spiralizing is an excellent way to introduce more root vegetables and squashes into your high raw diet to add to salads and replace cooked wheat pastas and noodles. Use this innovative technique freely to add a touch of creativity to your plant-based meals.

Elevate Your Raw Food Preparation Skills

Mastering healthy raw food preparation techniques is a vital aspect of thriving on a high raw plant-based diet. Dehydration, sun drying, food processing, blending, and spiralizing offer a wide range of possibilities for creating delicious, nutrient-dense raw dishes.

By understanding these methods and experimenting with various ingredients, textures, and flavors, you can craft raw meals that not only support your well-being but also delight your palate. Embrace the art of raw food preparation, and let your culinary creativity flourish.

Section References:

1. Barrett, D. M., Beaulieu, J. C., & Shewfelt, R. (2010). Color, flavor, texture, and nutritional quality of fresh-cut fruits and vegetables: desirable levels, instrumental and sensory measurement, and the effects of processing. Critical Reviews in Food Science and Nutrition, 50(5), 369-389.
2. Marathe, S. A., & Rajalakshmi, V. (2017). Solar drying of fruits and vegetables - A comprehensive review. Renewable and Sustainable Energy Reviews, 93, 789-796.
3. Raw Food Chef Certification Manual (n.d.). Living Light Culinary

Institute.
4. Selvan, P. S., & Haridas Rao, P. (2012). Physico-chemical changes in food during sun drying. Food Engineering Reviews, 4(1), 1-15.
5. Shalini, R., & Gupta, R. K. (2010). Nutrient retention in foods after legume-based curry preparation using common household methods. International Journal of Food Sciences and Nutrition, 61(7), 729-745.

EATING OUT: NAVIGATING RESTAURANTS, SOCIAL GATHERINGS, AND TRAVEL

Transitioning to a high raw plant-based diet doesn't mean you have to give up the pleasure of dining out, enjoying social gatherings, or exploring new culinary experiences while traveling.

With a few strategies and a proactive approach, you can maintain your commitment to a raw plant-based lifestyle while partaking in these activities. In this section, we'll explore how to navigate restaurants, social gatherings, and travel while staying true to your dietary choices.

Special Ordering at Restaurants

When dining out at restaurants that may not have raw plant-based options readily available on their menu, don't hesitate to request special accommodations. Many establishments are willing to accommodate dietary preferences and restrictions.

Here's how to navigate the restaurant experience when on a raw plant-based diet:

- **Review the Menu:** Start by examining the restaurant's menu online, if available. Look for salads, vegetable sides, and fruit-based options that may already align with your high raw diet.
- **Call Ahead:** Before making a reservation or arriving at the restaurant, consider calling ahead to inquire about their willingness to accommodate raw dietary preferences. Speak with the chef or manager to discuss possible menu modifications. Do your best to ask for meals containing raw foods the restaurant already has in stock.
- **Customize Your Order:** Once at the restaurant, communicate your dietary requirements clearly to your server. Ask for

modifications like extra vegetables, raw toppings, or simply requesting dishes to be prepared without cooking or oil.

- **Embrace Sides and Appetizers:** If the restaurant doesn't offer a raw entrée, consider ordering a variety of sides and appetizers like mixed greens, raw vegetable platters, or fresh fruit to create a satisfying meal.
- **Dressings and Sauces:** Be mindful of dressings and sauces, as they often contain cooked or processed ingredients. Request simple olive oil and lemon juice for salads, or ask for sauces to be served on the side so you can avoid them.
- **Be Patient and Grateful:** Remember that not all restaurants may be familiar with raw plant-based diets, so approach the situation with patience and gratitude. A courteous attitude can go a long way in receiving the cooperation of the staff.

Bringing Your Own Raw Food

In some cases, especially at potlucks, gatherings or events away from home where the menu options are limited, bringing your own raw food can be a practical and enjoyable solution so that you can still participate comfortably while maintaining your healthful dietary integrity.

Here are some tips for successfully incorporating your homemade raw dishes into your remote dining experience:

- **Plan Ahead:** If you know you'll be attending an event or gathering where raw options may be scarce, plan in advance by preparing raw dishes that are both delicious and visually appealing.
- **Portable Dishes:** Choose dishes that are easy to transport, such as raw salads, vegetable rolls, or fruit platters. Invest in portable containers or bento boxes to keep your food fresh during transport.
- **Share the Bounty:** Sharing your raw creations with others can be a great conversation starter and an opportunity to introduce friends and family to the delights of raw cuisine. Be prepared to share your recipes if others show interest.
- **Communicate Your Needs:** If you're attending an event, let the host or organizer know about your dietary preferences in advance. They may appreciate your proactive approach and even be willing to accommodate your needs.

Navigating Social Gatherings

Social gatherings, whether they're family celebrations, work events, or parties with friends, often revolve around food. Here's how to gracefully navigate these situations while staying true to your high raw plant-based diet:

- **Communicate in Advance:** If you're comfortable, communicate your dietary preferences to the host ahead of time. This allows them to plan accordingly and possibly include raw plant-based options.
- **Eat Beforehand:** To ensure you don't go hungry, eat a small, satisfying meal or snack before attending a gathering. This can help you resist the temptation of non-raw options.
- **BYORF (Bring Your Own Raw Food):** As mentioned earlier, consider bringing a raw dish to share. This not only ensures you have something to eat but also introduces others to raw cuisine.
- **Choose Wisely:** When at the gathering, scan the available options and choose raw-friendly items, such as fresh fruit, raw vegetable platters, or salads. Avoid sauces and dishes that are heavily cooked or processed.
- **Stay Social:** Focus on the social aspect of the gathering rather than solely on the food. Engage in conversations, connect with others, and enjoy the company.

Eating Raw While Traveling

Traveling as a high raw plant-based enthusiast may seem challenging at first, but you can transform that experience into an exciting adventure with some thoughtful preparation. Here are tips for maintaining your dietary choices while on the road:

- **Research Dining Options:** Before your trip, research restaurants and eateries at your destination that offer raw or vegan options. Websites, apps, and online reviews can be valuable resources.
- **Pack Raw Snacks:** Carry portable raw snacks like dried fruits, nuts, and seeds to keep you fueled between meals and during transit.
- **Seek Local Markets:** Explore local farmer's markets and grocery stores at your destination to stock up on fresh produce and raw ingredients for homemade meals.
- **Hotel Amenities:** If you're staying in a hotel, check if they offer in-room refrigerators. This can be handy for storing any fresh fruits or vegetables you bring with you.
- **Communication is Key:** When dining at restaurants and hotels

during your travels, clearly communicate your dietary preferences to the staff, and ask about menu options that align with your high raw diet.

Conclusion: Empowerment Through Preparation

Navigating restaurants, social gatherings, and travel while adhering to a high raw plant-based diet is entirely feasible with the right strategies. Whether you're special ordering at a restaurant, bringing your own raw food, or participating in social events, effective communication, preparation, and a positive attitude are your allies.

By approaching these situations proactively and with confidence, you can maintain your commitment to your healthful dietary choices while savoring the richness of life's culinary experiences.

Section References:

1. Forestell, C. A., & Spaeth, A. M. (2019). The neuroscience of mindful eating: Integrating the mind and body into the understanding of the biology of nutrition. In Mindfulness-Based Eating Awareness Training (MB-EAT) (pp. 27-36). Springer.
2. Radnitz, C., Beezhold, B., & DiMatteo, J. (2015). Investigation of lifestyle choices of individuals following a vegan diet for health and ethical reasons. Appetite, 90, 31-36.
3. Barnes, K. E., & Ball, L. (2017). Describing the eating behaviors of people who follow a vegan diet for ethical reasons. Appetite, 116, 225-230.
4. Lea, E., & Worsley, A. (2003). Benefits and barriers to the consumption of a vegetarian diet in Australia. Public Health Nutrition, 6(5), 505-511.

UNDERSTANDING AND OVERCOMING CHALLENGES

Embarking on a high raw plant-based diet is a transformative journey toward optimal health and well-being. However, like any significant change in lifestyle, it can come with its fair share of challenges, including nutrient deficiencies and cravings during the transition process.

Understanding the root causes of any cravings, addressing potential nutrient deficiencies, navigating transitional periods effectively and comfortably, and troubleshooting any additional issues that can arise are essential steps in successfully adopting and maintaining a high raw plant-based diet.

In this comprehensive section, we'll delve into the complexities of food cravings, explore how certain nutrient deficiencies may play a role, discuss die-off reactions related to gut flora, and provide insights into using transitional faux animal product foods as a temporary strategy during a shift from an unhealthy diet high in animal products.

Food Cravings

The Nature of Food Cravings

Food cravings are a common experience, and they can range from mild to intense. Understanding the underlying causes of these cravings is crucial for managing them effectively, especially when transitioning to a high raw plant-based diet. Here are some factors that contribute to food cravings:

- **Psychological Triggers:** Emotional states, stress, boredom, and even nostalgia can trigger food cravings. People often turn to familiar comfort foods in times of distress.
- **Habitual Patterns:** Long-standing dietary habits and routines can lead to cravings for familiar foods. Transitioning away from these

patterns can trigger cravings for the old diet.

- **Nutrient Deficiencies:** Cravings can sometimes signal nutrient deficiencies. For instance, a craving for sweets may indicate a need for magnesium, while a craving for salty foods may suggest a sodium or mineral deficiency.
- **Gut Microbiota:** The composition of your gut microbiota can influence food cravings. Unhealthy gut flora can lead to cravings for processed and sugary foods, as certain harmful bacteria thrive on these substances.

Cravings for Cooked Foods

If you are accustomed for mainly consuming cooked foods, it is natural to have occasional cravings for them. Here's how to address these cravings:

- **Transition Period:** Understand that cravings for cooked foods can be part of the transition. They often diminish over time as your palate adjusts to raw flavors.
- **Healthy Alternatives:** Opt for healthier alternatives to cooked comfort foods. Explore creative raw recipes that mimic familiar cooked dishes, such as raw vegetable lasagna or zucchini noodles with tomato sauce.
- **Mindful Eating:** Practice mindful eating by savoring each bite of your raw meals. Focus on the flavors, textures, and the nourishment that raw foods provide.
- **Stay Inspired:** Keep your enthusiasm for raw cuisine alive by trying new recipes, experimenting with different ingredients, and following raw food bloggers and chefs for inspiration.

Fortunately, as the many health benefits of enjoying a high raw plant-based diet start to become evident in your life, your desire to consume cooked foods will probably diminish over time.

Addressing Cravings

Cravings can be an indication that your body is trying to communicate its nutritional needs. When transitioning to a high raw plant-based diet, it's essential to pay attention to these signals and address them appropriately. Here's how to manage cravings and potential nutrient deficiencies:

- **Balanced Diet:** Ensure that your high raw plant-based diet is well-balanced and includes a variety of fruits, vegetables, nuts, seeds, and legumes. Diversifying your food choices can help meet your nutritional needs.

- **Hydration:** Sometimes, dehydration can be mistaken for hunger or cravings. Ensure you're staying adequately hydrated throughout the day by drinking plenty of water.
- **Monitor Nutrient Intake:** Track your dietary intake to ensure you're meeting your nutritional requirements. Consider consulting with a registered dietitian who specializes in plant-based nutrition to identify and address any potential deficiencies. For self-help, you can visit websites like www.cronometer.com to enter your food and drink intake in detail to assure you are covering all necessary nutritional bases with your raw plant-based diet.
- **Craving Substitutes:** When cravings strike, opt for healthier substitutes. For example, if you're craving sweets, reach for fresh fruits like berries, dates, or mangoes, which provide natural sweetness along with vitamins and minerals.
- **Supplements:** In some cases, supplements may be necessary to address specific nutrient deficiencies that can give rise to cravings, especially during the transition period. Common supplements for those on a high raw plant-based diet include vitamin B12 from microbes and vitamin D3 from lichen. A source of iron could also benefit menstruating women. You can also consider taking a good source of omega-3 fatty acids like algal oil derived from marine algae if your conversion of ALA contained in walnuts and flax and hemp seeds into EPA and DHA happens to be poor and you become forgetful as a result.

Gut Flora Die-Off (Herxheimer) Reactions

Navigating Die-off Reactions

As you transition to a high raw plant-based diet, it's not uncommon to experience die-off reactions in your gut flora. Known medically as a Herxheimer reaction, this is an entirely natural response to the destruction of harmful bacteria and other threatening microorganisms

When undergoing a dietary change to a raw plant-based diet, these reactions often occur as harmful bacteria and yeast colonies die and diminish in response to the absence of their preferred fuel sources, which are often found in processed and cooked foods, as well as in animal products.

The death of these organisms can release toxic substances that may make you briefly feel a bit ill, almost as if you have the flu, as your gut flora die-off detoxification process progresses.

Die-off reactions can also manifest as temporary discomfort, including bloating, gas, and changes in bowel habits. While navigating this brief dietary transition process should take no longer than about a week, here's some tips on how to best navigate these reactions for minimal discomfort:

- **Gradual Transition:** Consider a gradual transition to a high raw plant-based diet to minimize die-off reactions. Slowly reducing processed and cooked foods while increasing raw plant-based options can help your gut adjust.
- **Probiotics:** Incorporating probiotic-rich foods like sauerkraut, kimchi, and kombucha can support the growth of beneficial gut bacteria, helping to rebalance your microbiome.
- **Hydration and Fiber:** Drink plenty of water and consume fiber-rich raw foods like fruits, leafy green vegetables, and flaxseeds to support healthy digestion and flush out toxins.
- **Rest and Relaxation:** Stress can exacerbate die-off reactions. Incorporate stress-reduction techniques like meditation, deep breathing, or yoga into your routine to support your body during this transition.
- **Consult a Professional:** If die-off reactions persist or are severe, it may be helpful to consult with a healthcare professional or registered dietitian experienced in plant-based nutrition for personalized guidance.

Using Transition Faux Animal Product Foods Temporarily

For some individuals, especially those transitioning from a diet heavily reliant on animal products, incorporating transitional faux animal product foods can provide a bridge to a high raw plant-based diet.

These foods mimic the taste and texture of meat, cheese, milk and eggs but are made purely from plant-based ingredients. While they are generally not raw or part of a healthful diet due to their heavily-processed nature, they can help ease the transition and satisfy old dietary habits temporarily. Here's how to use them effectively:

- **Temporary Strategy:** Treat faux meat foods as a transitional strategy rather than a long-term dietary staple. Use them sparingly as you gradually increase your intake of raw fruits, vegetables, nuts, and seeds.

- **Read Labels:** Choose faux animal products that contain minimal processed ingredients and additives. Look for options made from whole, recognizable plant-based ingredients.
- **Balanced Meals:** When incorporating faux animal foods, balance them with a variety of raw plant-based foods to ensure you're still receiving the full spectrum of nutrients.
- **Experiment with Whole Foods:** As you become more comfortable with your high raw diet, experiment with whole, unprocessed plant-based protein sources like legumes, nuts, seeds, and sprouted grains to replace faux animal product options.

Remember that transition foods are generally not health foods, so be sure to make your use of them as minimal and brief as possible to help you progress more quickly on your nutritional healing journey using raw plant foods.

Troubleshooting a Raw Plant-Based Diet

Transitioning to a high raw plant-based diet can be a rewarding journey, but it's not uncommon to encounter certain common challenges along the way. From digestion issues to social situations, troubleshooting common roadblocks can help you stay committed to your health and dietary goals.

While we have already mentioned many ways to troubleshoot issues that can arises when transitioning to and maintaining a raw plant-based diet, this section will summarize and explore in greater detail some common challenges faced by individuals on a high raw plant-based diet and provide practical solutions you can use to overcome them.

Digestive Discomfort

One of the most common issues when transitioning to a high raw plant-based diet is digestive discomfort. This can manifest as bloating, gas, or changes in bowel habits. These challenges often arise as your body adapts to increased fiber intake and the unique characteristics of raw foods. Here's some tips on how to troubleshoot digestive discomfort you may initially experience when transitioning to a raw plant-based diet:

- **Gradual Transition:** Slowly increase your intake of raw foods, allowing your digestive system time to adapt. Start with easily digestible fruits and vegetables and gradually incorporate more complex raw dishes.

- **Hydration:** Ensure you're drinking enough water throughout the day to support the digestion of fiber-rich foods. Hydration can help prevent constipation and promote smoother digestion.
- **Chew Thoroughly:** Take your time to chew your food thoroughly. Chewing breaks down food into smaller particles, making it easier for your stomach and intestines to process.
- **Probiotics:** Consider incorporating probiotic-rich foods like sauerkraut, kimchi, and kombucha into your diet to support a healthy gut microbiome and improve digestion.
- **Digestive Enzymes:** Some individuals may benefit from digestive enzyme supplements, especially during the transition period. Consult with a healthcare professional or registered dietitian for personalized guidance.

Social and Cultural Challenges

Maintaining a high raw plant-based diet in social and cultural contexts can be challenging, as many social gatherings and traditional dishes are centered around cooked foods. Here's some tips for how to navigate these situations:

- **Communication:** Communicate your dietary preferences politely but assertively to friends and family. Explain the health benefits of your chosen diet to help others understand your choices.
- **Contribute to Potlucks:** When attending potlucks or gatherings, offer to bring a raw plant-based dish to share. This ensures you have a suitable option to enjoy and introduces others to raw cuisine based solely on plant foods.
- **Flexibility:** Be open to making exceptions on rare occasions, especially when visiting friends or family who may not be familiar with or accommodating of your dietary choices. Focus on the overall balance of your diet.
- **Seek Like-Minded Communities:** Connect with like-minded individuals through online communities, local meetups, or social media groups to find support and share experiences with others who follow a high raw diet.

Maintaining Nutritional Balance

Sustaining yourself well a well-balanced diet on a high raw plant-based lifestyle requires nutritional balance to meet your nutritional needs properly. Some individuals may worry about specific nutrient deficiencies. Here's how to ensure nutritional balance when on a raw plant-based diet:

- **Diverse Diet:** Aim for a diverse range of fruits, vegetables, nuts, seeds, and legumes to provide a wide spectrum of nutrients.
- **Supplementation:** Consider supplementing with nutrients that may be challenging to obtain from a high raw diet, such as vitamin B12, vitamin D, and omega-3 fatty acids. Consult with a healthcare professional for personalized recommendations.
- **Regular Check-ups:** Schedule regular check-ups and blood tests to monitor your nutrient levels. This can help you identify and address any deficiencies promptly.
- **Consult a Dietitian:** If you have concerns about your nutrient intake or require guidance on meal planning, consult with a registered dietitian who specializes in plant-based nutrition.

Protein Adequacy on a High Raw Plant-Based Diet

One of the most common concerns raised about a high raw plant-based diet is protein adequacy. However, it's important to understand that protein deficiency is generally not a concern as long as you are meeting your calorie needs with a variety of raw plant-based foods.

In fact, the World Health Organization (WHO), the Food and Agriculture Organization of the United Nations (FAO) and the United Nations University (UNU) have conducted a joint study based on extensive research into protein requirements. The study has definitively established relatively low recommendations for dietary protein intake for humans.

The WHO's research has shown that even in populations with relatively low protein intake, protein deficiency is exceptionally rare. This is because most plant-based foods, such as fruits, greens, vegetables, nuts, seeds, and legumes, contain some amount of protein. When you consume a well-balanced high raw plant-based diet that is calorically adequate and includes a variety of these foods, you can easily meet your protein needs.

Furthermore, focusing on calorie intake is crucial. When you consume enough calories from raw plant-based sources, you naturally obtain sufficient protein to support your body's daily requirements. It's worth noting that while individual protein requirements may vary based on factors such as age, sex, pregnancy status, and activity level, the protein content in raw plant-based foods is generally adequate for most individuals.

By prioritizing a diverse and calorie-sufficient high raw plant-based diet, you can confidently enjoy the many health benefits that this lifestyle offers without undue concern about protein deficiency. Remember that it's always a good idea to consult with a healthcare professional or registered dietitian who specializes in plant-based nutrition to ensure that you are meeting your individual dietary needs.

Sustainability Concerns

Some individuals with a high sensitivity to environmental issues and the footprint of their lives may have concerns about the environmental impact and sustainability of a high raw plant-based diet. Here's some ideas for how to address such concerns:

- **Local and Seasonal Foods:** Choose locally grown and seasonal produce whenever possible to reduce your carbon footprint.
- **Reducing Food Waste:** Minimize food waste by planning your meals, storing ingredients properly, and using all parts of fruits and vegetables, including peels and stems, in creative recipes and smoothies. Also, be sure to compost any raw food waste and use it to fertilize your own food garden or a plot in a community garden.
- **Educate Yourself:** Stay informed about the environmental impact of various foods and agricultural practices. Knowledge empowers you to make sustainable choices within your dietary preferences.
- **Advocacy:** Consider advocating for sustainable farming practices and supporting initiatives that promote ethical and environmentally friendly agriculture.

Choose Empowering Solutions

Transitioning to a high raw plant-based diet is a transformative and empowering journey that may come with its share of challenges. Remember to embrace the power of whole, raw plant-based foods, and trust in the nourishing and healthful journey you've embarked upon as you resolve to overcome such issues as they arise.

Know that by understanding the factors that contribute to cravings, addressing potential nutrient deficiencies, and navigating transitional periods with patience and grace, you can readily surmount any obstacles on your path to optimal health and vitality.

Remember that troubleshooting the common challenges that can arise on a high raw plant-based diet effectively is essential for long-term success on this healthful and natural dietary journey, so do not avoid doing this work.

By addressing digestive discomfort, navigating social and cultural situations, maintaining nutritional balance, managing cravings for cooked foods and animal products, and addressing sustainability concerns, you can empower yourself to embrace the many benefits of a high raw plant-based lifestyle.

Since everyone's journey in life is unique, make sure to apply your patience, perseverance, and creativity to your personal dietary situation to learn how to thrive on this natural and empowering path to greater health and well-being.

Chapter References:

1. Gibson, G. R., Hutkins, R., Sanders, M. E., Prescott, S. L., Reimer, R. A., Salminen, S. J., ... & Reid, G. (2017). Expert consensus document: The International Scientific Association for Probiotics and Prebiotics (ISAPP) consensus statement on the definition and scope of prebiotics. Nature Reviews Gastroenterology & Hepatology, 14(8), 491-502.
2. Smith, A. P., & Rogers, P. J. (1995). Psychological stress and the human immune system: A meta-analytic study of 30 years of inquiry. Psychological Bulletin, 130(4), 601-630.
3. Michener, W., Rozin, P., Freeman, E., & Gale, N. (1991). The role of lowfat flavor in dietary restraint, mood and internal state. Physiology & Behavior, 50(3), 474-480.
4. Lin, M. J., Dai, X. Y., Ding, H. B., & Zhong, H. (2019). The role of gut microbiota in the effects of maternal obesity during pregnancy on offspring metabolism. Bioscience Reports, 39(1), BSR20181319.
5. Chassaing, B., Gewirtz, A. T., & Ley, R. E. (2014). Intestinal epithelial cell toll-like receptor 5 regulates the intestinal microbiota to prevent low-grade inflammation and metabolic syndrome in mice. Gastroenterology, 147(6), 1363-1377.
6. De Filippo, C., Cavalieri, D., Di Paola, M., Ramazzotti, M., Poullet, J. B., Massart, S., ... & Lionetti, P. (2010). Impact of diet in shaping gut microbiota revealed by a comparative study in children from Europe and rural Africa. Proceedings of the National Academy of Sciences, 107(33), 14691-14696.
7. Protein and Amino Acid Requirements in Human Nutrition: Report of a Joint FAO/WHO/UNU Expert Consultation. URL: https://iris.who.int/bitstream/handle/10665/43411/WHO_TRS_935_eng.pdf

94

PART IV: PUTTING IT ALL TOGETHER

CREATING YOUR PERSONALIZED NUTRITIONAL HEALING PLAN

Embarking on a high raw plant-based diet is a transformative nutritional healing journey towards health and vitality. To harness the full benefits of this healthier and kinder lifestyle, it's essential to develop a personalized nutritional plan that aligns with your unique needs and goals.

This section will guide you through the process of creating a tailored nutritional plan for your unique situation, offering strategies for both the transition and maintenance phases of your high raw plant-based journey.

Understanding Your Overall Nutritional Plan

A nutritional plan, often referred to as a meal plan or dietary plan, is a structured approach to how you consume food to meet your nutritional requirements, preferences, and health objectives.

For a high raw plant-based diet, your nutritional plan will outline the types and quantities of raw plant foods you intend to incorporate regularly. Here's how to create a comprehensive plan tailored to your specific needs:

Define Your Dietary Goals

Begin by clarifying your dietary objectives. What are your aspirations with a high raw plant-based diet? Common goals include weight management, increased energy, improved digestion, enhanced mental clarity, and overall well-being. Identifying your specific goals will serve as the foundation for shaping your nutritional plan.

Calculate Your Caloric Needs

To ensure you meet your daily energy requirements, calculate your caloric needs based on factors such as age, sex, pregnancy and menstruation status, activity level, and health objectives. Numerous online tools and calculators can assist you in determining an appropriate caloric intake, such as www.cronometer.com.

Plan Your Macronutrient Ratios

Consider the macronutrient ratios that align with your dietary goals, although the precise ratios may vary based on your objectives.

A general guideline for a high raw plant-based diet is approximately 70-80% of calories from carbohydrates, 10-15% from fats, and 10-15% from proteins. You can adjust these ratios somewhat according to your individual dietary needs and healing requirements.

Select a Variety of Whole, Raw Plant Foods

Emphasize whole, raw plant foods in your dietary plan that complement your macronutrient ratios and dietary objectives.

This category should ideally include a dominating amount of fruits and leafy greens, with the addition in lesser amounts of other vegetables, nuts, seeds, legumes, and sprouted grains.

To ensure that you include a broad spectrum of micronutrients, diversify your raw plant food choices, and incorporate a colorful array of fruits and vegetables.

Construct Balanced Meals

Design balanced meals that encompass a variety of raw foods. Breakfast might center on a colorful fruit salad, while a typical heavier afternoon meal might consist of a generous salad with leafy greens, colorful vegetables, nuts, seeds, and a dressing crafted from ingredients like avocado or raw tahini. A light dinner could include a fruit-based smoothie or a raw soup to introduce some variety into your diet.

Consider Meal Timing

Tailor your meal timing pattern to your preferences and energy levels.

While some individuals thrive on three larger meals a day, others may prefer several smaller meals and snacks. Tune in to your body's cues and adjust your meal timing accordingly.

Prioritize Hydration

Remember to stay well-hydrated throughout the day by including spring water as well as water-rich fruits, greens and vegetables in your meals. Adequate hydration supports digestion and overall well-being, and it remains a critical benefit of consuming a high raw plant-based lifestyle.

Transition Period: Crafting Your Dietary Plan for Greater Health

During the transition to a high raw plant-based diet, creating a thoughtful plan can ease the adjustment process. Here are some constructive steps you can go through to craft a personalized transitional nutritional plan you can follow.

(1) Embark on a Gradual Transition

Initiate your nutritional healing journey by incrementally increasing the proportion of raw plant foods in your diet while reducing cooked or processed plant or animal foods. Begin with one raw meal a day and progressively incorporate more raw plant foods into your daily intake.

(2) Experiment with Raw Recipes

Explore a variety of raw plant food recipes and dishes to identify those you enjoy most and that seem most suitable for your health-enhancing goals.

You can start off with simple recipes like smoothie bowls, salads, and fruit platters. As you become more adept at raw preparations, you can start to venture into more complex dishes to expand your culinary repertoire.

(3) Monitor Your Progress

Maintain a food diary to track your dietary intake and assess how your body responds to the transition. Document any changes in energy levels, digestion, and overall well-being to fine-tune your plan.

Maintenance Period: Refining Your Plan

After successfully transitioning to a high raw plant-based lifestyle, you can refine your nutritional plan to support long-term well-being. Here are steps to further enhance your plan:

Regularly Review and Adapt

Periodically review your nutritional plan to ensure it aligns with your current dietary goals and lifestyle. As your needs and preferences evolve, your plan may require adjustments to remain effective.

Embrace Seasonal Eating

Celebrate seasonal variations in your diet. Embrace the abundance of fresh, seasonal fruits and vegetables available throughout the year. Seasonal eating not only enhances your culinary experience but also provides a diverse range of flavors and nutrients.

Explore Food Combining

Delve into food combining principles, such as proper fruit and greens pairing, to optimize digestion and nutrient absorption. Food combining can enhance your high raw plant-based experience by promoting better digestion and reducing discomfort.

Periodic Detoxification

Consider incorporating periodic detoxification or cleansing phases into your plan. These intervals may involve short periods of consuming exclusively raw foods to reset your body, promote detoxification, and reinvigorate your commitment to health.

Consult a Professional

If you encounter specific health concerns or dietary inquiries, seek guidance from a registered dietitian or nutritionist who specializes in plant-based nutrition. Their expertise can provide personalized recommendations and help you fine-tune your nutritional plan to address your unique needs.

Thriving on Your High Raw Journey

Creating a personalized nutritional plan is a pivotal step in maximizing the benefits of a high raw plant-based lifestyle. Whether you are in the transition phase or maintaining your dietary choices, remember that your plan should evolve in alignment with your goals, preferences, and health requirements. Relish the diversity and vibrancy of raw plant foods, heed your body's signals, and cherish the path to optimal health and well-being.

TRACKING PROGRESS: THE IMPORTANCE OF KEEPING A FOOD JOURNAL

Starting your high raw plant-based dietary journey is a powerful step towards vibrant health and well-being. To navigate this path effectively and make the most of your transition and maintenance phases, consider the invaluable tool of a food journal.

In this section, we will explore what a food journal is, why it is crucial for your high raw plant-based lifestyle, and how to create and maintain one tailored to your unique needs.

Understanding the Role of Food Journals

A food journal, sometimes also referred to as a food diary or nutrition journal, is a written record of your daily dietary intake.

A food journal serves as a comprehensive snapshot of what you eat and drink, including portion sizes, meal timings, and any accompanying thoughts or emotions related to your food choices.

Many nutritionists require their clients to keep an accurate food journal so that they can better assess precisely where your diet needs adjustment.

Why Keep a Food Journal?

While the idea of documenting your meals may seem simple, the benefits of maintaining a food journal for a high raw plant-based diet are profound. They include:

- **Enhanced Self-Awareness:** A food journal encourages mindful eating by prompting you to pay closer attention to your food choices. It heightens your awareness of what you consume and helps you recognize patterns in your dietary habits.

- **Goal Tracking:** It provides a visual record of your dietary progress, making it easier to track your adherence to a high raw plant-based diet. You can see your journey unfold, celebrate successes, and identify areas for improvement.
- **Identification of Triggers:** Food journals can help you pinpoint triggers for overeating or emotional eating. By recording your feelings and circumstances surrounding each meal, you can uncover connections between your emotions and eating habits.
- **Nutritional Analysis:** You can assess your nutrient intake, ensuring you meet your daily requirements for essential nutrients like vitamins, minerals, and macronutrients (carbohydrates, fats, and proteins).
- **Accountability:** Maintaining a food journal fosters accountability. Knowing that you will record your choices may motivate you to make more health-conscious decisions.
- **Problem-Solving:** When faced with challenges or setbacks, reviewing your food journal can help you identify the root causes of issues and find effective solutions. It becomes a valuable tool for troubleshooting and making informed adjustments to your dietary plan.

Creating Your Food Journal

Now that you understand why food journals are so helpful to your success in a nutritional healing process, let's delve into how to create and maintain one that aligns with your high raw plant-based lifestyle.

To create a meaningful food journal, you can follow these steps:

1. Choose Your Journal Format
Select a journal format that suits your preferences and lifestyle. You can use a physical notebook, a digital app, or even a simple spreadsheet. The key is to find a format that you are comfortable with and will consistently use.

2. Set Clear Objectives
Before you start, establish clear objectives for your food journal. What do you hope to achieve by keeping one? This might include tracking your raw food intake, identifying potential food sensitivities, or monitoring your energy levels throughout the day.

3. Record Each Meal and Snack
For each meal and snack, record the following details:

- Date and time of the meal.
- Description of the foods and beverages consumed, including ingredients and preparation methods.
- Portion sizes or approximate quantities.
- Any condiments or seasonings used.
- Your emotional state before and after eating.

4. Note Emotional and Physical Cues

Pay attention to any emotional or physical cues related to your meals. Did you eat because you were hungry, stressed, bored, or influenced by external factors? How did you feel after eating? Recording these cues can help uncover emotional eating patterns.

5. Include Daily Notes

Use your food journal to jot down any additional daily notes related to your high raw plant-based journey. This might include reflections on your energy levels, cravings, digestion, or any challenges you encountered.

6. Reflect and Analyze

Regularly review your food journal to analyze your dietary habits. Look for patterns in your eating behavior and identify areas where you excel or need improvement. Are there certain times of day or situations that trigger specific food choices?

7. Celebrate Achievements and Set Goals

Celebrate your successes along the way. Acknowledge achievements, whether it's sticking to your raw food goals, overcoming cravings, or experiencing improved well-being. Use your food journal as a source of motivation.

8. Adjust Your Plan

As you gain insights from your food journal, be open to adjusting your high raw plant-based plan. If you notice that certain foods consistently make you feel better or worse, make informed adjustments to your dietary choices.

9. Stay Consistent

Consistency is key. Make it a habit to record your meals and snacks promptly. The more consistently you maintain your food journal, the more valuable insights you'll gather.

10. Seek Support

Consider sharing your food journal with a trusted friend, family member, or a healthcare professional who specializes in plant-based nutrition. They can provide guidance, offer insights, and support your dietary goals.

A Food Journal is a Valuable Companion on Your Journey

Overall, a food journal serves as a powerful companion on your high raw plant-based journey. It enhances self-awareness, aids in goal tracking, and facilitates the identification of triggers and solutions.

By creating and maintaining a personalized food journal, you can optimize your transition to a high raw plant-based lifestyle and reap the numerous benefits it offers.

Section References:

1. Hollis, J. F., Gullion, C. M., Stevens, V. J., Brantley, P. J., Appel, L. J., Ard, J. D., ... & Svetkey, L. P. (2008). Weight loss during the intensive intervention phase of the weight-loss maintenance trial. American Journal of Preventive Medicine, 35(2), 118-126. This study emphasizes the importance of keeping a food journal in achieving and maintaining weight loss goals.
2. Butryn, M. L., Phelan, S., Hill, J. O., & Wing, R. R. (2007). Consistent self-monitoring of weight: a key component of successful weight loss maintenance. Obesity, 15(12), 3091-3096. The research highlights the role of self-monitoring, including food journaling, in the long-term success of weight management.
3. Kristeller, J. L., & Hallett, C. B. (1999). An exploratory study of a meditation-based intervention for binge eating disorder. Journal of Health Psychology, 4(3), 357-363. This study examines the positive impact of mindfulness-based approaches, which include food journaling, on managing binge eating disorder.
4. Boutelle, K. N., Kuckertz, J. M., Carlson, J., & Amir, N. (2014). A pilot study evaluating a one-session attention modification training to decrease overeating in obese children. Appetite, 76, 180-185. The research discusses the potential of mindful eating practices, like food journaling, in reducing overeating behaviors in children.
5. Tomiyama, A. J., Mann, T., Vinas, D., Hunger, J. M., Dejager, J., & Taylor, S. E. (2010). Low calorie dieting increases cortisol. Psychosomatic Medicine, 72(4), 357-364. This study highlights the importance of mindful eating and the potential pitfalls of extreme dieting, which can be monitored through food journaling.
6. Burrows, T. L., Martin, R. J., & Collins, C. E. (2010). A systematic review of the validity of dietary assessment methods in children when compared with the method of doubly labeled water. Journal of the

American Dietetic Association, 110(10), 1501-1510. A systematic review that discusses the validity of different dietary assessment methods, including food journaling, in children.

7. Fogelholm, M. (2010). Physical activity, fitness and fatness: relations to mortality, morbidity and disease risk factors. A systematic review. Obesity Reviews, 11(3), 202-221. This systematic review explores the relationship between dietary records and various health outcomes, including mortality and disease risk factors.

8. Johansson, L., Solvoll, K., & Bjørneboe, G. E. (1998). Drevon CA. Under-and overreporting of energy intake related to weight status and lifestyle in a nationwide sample. American Journal of Clinical Nutrition, 68(2), 266-274. The study investigates the prevalence of underreporting and overreporting of energy intake in dietary records and its relation to weight status.

9. Howe, G. R., & Blackadar, C. B. (1981). Dietary intake of vitamins and minerals in Ontario. American Journal of Epidemiology, 113(2), 215-227. An example of a study assessing dietary intake of vitamins and minerals using food records, highlighting the value of such records in nutritional research.

10. Thompson, F. E., & Byers, T. (1994). Dietary assessment resource manual. Journal of Nutrition, 124(11), 2245S-2317S. This comprehensive resource provides guidance on dietary assessment methods, including food records, and their applications in nutritional research.

BUILDING A SUPPORTIVE FOOD ENVIRONMENT

Embarking on a high raw plant-based dietary journey is not just about changing what you eat; it's about creating an environment that supports your new lifestyle.

In this section, we'll explore the importance of a supportive food environment and provide practical guidance on how to garner support from friends and family, make behavioral changes within your home, and successfully transition to a high raw plant-based diet.

The Importance of a Supportive Food Environment

Your surroundings significantly influence your dietary choices. A supportive food environment can make your transition to a high raw plant-based diet smoother and more sustainable.

Here are some key reasons why it matters to build a supportive food environment around you to help ensure your success in following a high raw plant-based diet:

- **Reduced Temptations:** A supportive environment minimizes the presence of unhealthy, cooked, or processed foods that might tempt you away from your raw plant-based goals.
- **Increased Motivation:** When your home and social circles align with your dietary values, you're more motivated to stay on track and make positive choices.
- **Accountability:** Sharing your goals with supportive individuals creates accountability, as they can encourage and motivate you on your journey.
- **Positive Reinforcement:** Surrounding yourself with like-minded

individuals reinforces the benefits of your dietary choices, making it easier to stay committed.

Practical Strategies to Create a Supportive Food Environment

Now, let's delve into some practical strategies you can use to build and maintain a supportive food environment:

Communicate Your Goals

Start by sharing your dietary goals and reasons for adopting a high raw plant-based diet with your friends and family. Open and honest communication is key to garnering their support. Explain how this dietary shift aligns with your health and wellness objectives.

Seek Like-Minded Allies

Identify individuals in your social circles who share similar dietary preferences or health-conscious attitudes. These allies can be your sources of support, understanding, and inspiration. Join online or local plant-based communities to connect with like-minded individuals.

Family Participation

Encourage family members to join you on your high raw plant-based journey, even if only partially. You can involve them in meal planning and preparation to foster a sense of shared responsibility. Engage in open discussions about how this dietary shift can benefit the entire family.

Remove Temptations

In your home environment, gradually eliminate cooked and processed foods, as well as cooking implements that may no longer serve your dietary goals. Donate or store non-compliant items to create a clear distinction between your old and new food choices.

Stock Up on Raw Essentials

Ensure your kitchen is well-stocked with raw essentials such as fresh fruits, vegetables, nuts, seeds, and sprouted grains. Having readily available raw options makes it easier to prepare nourishing meals and snacks.

Meal Planning

Devote time to plan your meals in advance. Include a variety of raw recipes and dishes in your weekly meal plan to keep your diet interesting and satisfying. Explore new raw food preparation techniques and experiment with flavors.

Educate Your Support Network
Share informative resources, books, documentaries, or articles that highlight the health benefits of a high raw plant-based diet. Educating your support network can help them understand your choices and motivations better.

Encourage Respectful Dining
When dining out with friends or family, choose restaurants that offer raw or plant-based options. Communicate your dietary needs politely and in advance to ensure a pleasant dining experience for everyone.

Be Flexible and Patient
Understand that not everyone in your support network may fully embrace your dietary choices. Be patient and flexible in your interactions, and avoid imposing your beliefs on others. Focus on your own journey and lead by example.

Celebrate Successes Together
Celebrate milestones and achievements with your support network. Whether it's a successful week of raw eating or improved health markers, acknowledge and share your successes with those who support you.

Nurturing Your High Raw Plant-Based Journey

Building a supportive food environment is generally essential for your success in adopting a high raw plant-based diet when many other people around you may eat differently.

Through effective communication, education, and the removal of dietary temptations, you can create a space where your dietary choices are not only respected but also embraced.

Remember that surrounding yourself with supportive friends and family who share your goals will not only make your dietary healing journey more enjoyable but also enhance your chances of achieving optimal health and well-being.

Section References:

1. Nielsen, A. (2017). The Scandinavian 24-Hour Movement Guidelines for Children and Adolescents: An Integration of Physical Activity, Sedentary Behaviour, and Sleep. Scandinavian Journal of Medicine & Science in Sports, 27(12), 1811-1817. This study emphasizes the importance of a supportive environment, including family and peer

support, in promoting healthy behaviors in children and adolescents.

2. Dallacker, M., Hertwig, R., Peters, E., & Mata, J. (2016). Lower home cooking frequency and perceived barriers are associated with unhealthy eating in young adults. Public Health Nutrition, 19(3), 472-479. The research explores the impact of the home food environment on dietary choices and highlights the role of perceived barriers.

3. Liese, A. D., & Ma, X. (2015). Food store types, availability, and cost of foods in a rural environment. Journal of the American Dietetic Association, 105(3), 417-424. This study delves into the accessibility and affordability of healthy food options in different food store environments, shedding light on the importance of a supportive food environment.

4. Tang, J., Tang, L., & Tudor-Locke, C. (2018). How active are people in metropolitan areas? An observational study of physical activity distribution in Qingdao, China. BMC Public Health, 18(1), 725. The study examines the role of the built environment, including access to parks and recreational areas, in promoting physical activity, which can be extended to support a healthy diet.

5. Draper, C., & Lambert, E. V. (2012). A descriptive study of the diet and physical activity practices of secondary school students in the Northern Suburbs of Cape Town. South African Journal of Clinical Nutrition, 25(2), 67-74. This research investigates the influence of the home and school environments on the dietary and physical activity behaviors of adolescents.

6. Stok, F. M., de Vet, E., de Wit, J. B., Luszczynska, A., Safron, M., de Ridder, D. T., ... & Gaspar, T. (2016). The proof is in the eating: subjective peer norms are a causal factor in adolescents' eating behaviour. Appetite, 96, 160-165. The study examines the impact of peer norms and social environments on adolescents' eating behaviors, underlining the importance of a supportive social network.

7. Valanou, E., Bamia, C., Trichopoulou, A., Dangour, A. D., & Anastasiou, C. A. (2018). Dietary patterns and long-term survival: a systematic review and meta-analysis of prospective cohort studies. European Journal of Clinical Nutrition, 72(1), 15-23. A meta-analysis of prospective cohort studies that investigates the relationship between dietary patterns and long-term survival, highlighting the significance of a supportive dietary environment.

8. Blake, C. E., Wethington, E., Farrell, T. J., Bisogni, C. A., & Devine, C. M. (2011). Behavioral contexts, food-choice coping strategies, and dietary quality of a multiethnic sample of employed parents. Journal of the American Dietetic Association, 111(3), 401-407. This research explores the behavioral contexts and coping strategies related to food choices, emphasizing the role of the environment in dietary quality.

9. Ball, K., & Crawford, D. (2005). Socioeconomic status and weight change in adults: a review. Social Science & Medicine, 60(9), 1987-2010. The study reviews the impact of socioeconomic status and the food environment on weight change in adults, providing insights into the importance of a supportive environment in weight management.

10. Caspi, C. E., Sorensen, G., Subramanian, S. V., & Kawachi, I. (2012). The local food environment and diet: a systematic review. Health & Place, 18(5), 1172-1187. A systematic review that examines the relationship between the local food environment and dietary habits, underscoring the influence of environmental factors on food choices.

STAYING CONSISTENT AND MAINTAINING WELLNESS

Making the transition to a high raw plant-based diet is a significant step toward improved health and vitality. However, the journey doesn't end with the transition; it's essential to stay consistent and maintain your newfound wellness.

In this section, we will explore strategies for long-term consistency and how to thrive on a high raw plant-based diet while promoting overall wellness.

The Challenge of Maintaining Long-Term Consistency

Staying consistent on a high raw plant-based diet may present challenges, especially in a world where processed and cooked foods and animal products are abundant and readily available. However, with dedication and the right strategies, you can thrive on this dietary path for the long haul.

Some sensible tips for enhancing your long term dietary consistency to support your nutritional healing plan include:

Continuous Education

Stay informed and up-to-date about the benefits of a high raw plant-based diet. Keep learning about the nutritional value of various raw foods and the scientific evidence supporting this dietary approach. Understanding the positive impact on your health can motivate you to stay consistent.

Variety is Key

One way to ensure long-term adherence to a high raw plant-based diet is by maintaining variety in your meals. Experiment with different fruits, vegetables, nuts, seeds, and sprouted grains to keep your diet exciting and appealing. Diversity not only enhances your nutritional intake but also prevents dietary boredom.

Meal Planning and Preparation

Devote time to meal planning and preparation. Set aside specific days for grocery shopping, meal prepping, and batch-cooking raw staples like sprouted grains or raw nut butters. Having prepared raw ingredients on hand simplifies the process of creating satisfying meals.

Mindful Eating

Practice mindful eating to stay in tune with your body's hunger and satiety cues. Avoid distractions like television or screens while eating and savor the flavors, textures, and aromas of your raw meals. Mindful eating enhances your connection with food and can prevent overeating.

Social Support

Maintain connections with like-minded individuals who share your dietary values. Join local or online raw food communities, attend meetups, and engage in discussions with fellow enthusiasts. Social support can provide encouragement and a sense of belonging.

Regular Exercise

Incorporate regular physical activity into your routine. Exercise not only supports overall health but also complements your high raw plant-based diet by improving circulation, promoting detoxification, and enhancing your sense of well-being. Walking is a particularly natural and beneficial type of exercise you can incorporate into your lifestyle.

Mind-Body Practices

Explore mind-body practices such as yoga, meditation, or tai chi. These practices can help manage stress, improve mental clarity, and enhance your connection to your body, aligning with the holistic principles of a high raw plant-based lifestyle.

Set Realistic Goals

Set achievable goals for yourself on your raw food journey. Instead of aiming for perfection, focus on continuous improvement. Celebrate your successes, no matter how small, and learn from any challenges you encounter.

Periodic Detoxification

Consider incorporating periodic detoxification or cleansing protocols into your routine. These can help reset your digestive system, eliminate toxins, and revitalize your commitment to a high raw plant-based diet.

Seek Professional Guidance

If you encounter health concerns or challenges, seek guidance from healthcare, nutritionist or nutritional healer professionals experienced in plant-based nutrition and how to use it to improve your health. They can offer tailored advice, monitor your progress, and address any specific dietary or health-related issues.

Thriving on Your High Raw Plant-Based Journey

Staying consistent and maintaining wellness on a high raw plant-based diet is achievable with the right strategies and mindset. By continually educating yourself, maintaining variety, practicing mindful eating, and engaging with supportive communities, you can thrive in the long term.

Remember that wellness encompasses not only physical health but also mental and emotional well-being. By nurturing all aspects of your health, you can fully embrace the benefits of a high raw plant-based lifestyle.

Section References:

1. Fraser, G. E. (2009). Vegetarian diets: what do we know of their effects on common chronic diseases? The American Journal of Clinical Nutrition, 89(5), 1607S-1612S. This comprehensive review discusses the long-term health benefits of vegetarian diets, including high raw plant-based diets, in preventing chronic diseases.
2. Tuso, P. J., Ismail, M. H., Ha, B. P., & Bartolotto, C. (2013). Nutritional update for physicians: plant-based diets. The Permanente Journal, 17(2), 61-66. The article provides insights into the importance of maintaining a plant-based diet for long-term health and wellness, with a focus on variety and balanced nutrition.
3. Poulsen, S. K., Crone, C., Astrup, A., & Larsen, T. M. (2014). Long-term adherence to the New Nordic Diet and the effects on body weight, anthropometry, and blood pressure: a 12-month follow-up study. European Journal of Nutrition, 53(1), 147-157. This study

investigates the long-term adherence to a specific dietary pattern (New Nordic Diet) and its effects on various health markers, highlighting the significance of consistency.

4. O'Reilly, G. A., Cook, L., Spruijt-Metz, D., & Black, D. S. (2014). Mindfulness-based interventions for obesity-related eating behaviours: a literature review. Obesity Reviews, 15(6), 453-461. The review explores the role of mindfulness-based practices in promoting long-term consistency and healthy eating behaviors.

5. Vormund, K., Braun, J., Rohrmann, S., & Bopp, M. (2015). Impact of vegetarian diet on the risk of urinary tract infections in men: a Multicenter Case-Control Study. The Journal of Nutrition, Health & Aging, 19(2), 161-165. A study examining the impact of a long-term vegetarian diet on health outcomes, including the risk of urinary tract infections.

6. Van Dyke, N., & Drinkwater, E. J. (2010). Review article relationships between intuitive eating and health indicators: literature review. Public Health Nutrition, 13(10), 1207-1216. This literature review explores the connections between intuitive eating, long-term dietary consistency, and health indicators.

7. Ghosh, S., & Hewison, M. (2009). Vitamin D and the immune system: therapeutic potential in multiple sclerosis. Biochemical Society Transactions, 37(1), 137-142. Discusses the holistic approach to health, including the role of vitamin D in immune function and overall well-being.

8. Pratt, M., Sarmiento, O. L., Montes, F., Ogilvie, D., Marcus, B. H., Perez, L. G., ... & Matsudo, V. (2012). The implications of megatrends in information and communication technology and transportation for changes in global physical activity. The Lancet, 380(9838), 282-293. An examination of the importance of physical activity and its role in holistic well-being.

9. Boehm, J. K., Soo, J., & Zevon, E. S. (2018). Longitudinal associations between psychological well-being and the consumption of fruits and vegetables. Health Psychology, 37(10), 959-967. Investigates the connection between psychological well-being and dietary choices, emphasizing the holistic impact of a diet rich in fruits and vegetables.

10. Roberts, D. E. (2019). Is the juice worth the squeeze? The potential health benefits of functional foods. Environmental Health Perspectives, 127(2), 025001. This article highlights the potential health benefits of functional foods, which play a role in holistic well-being when incorporated into a high raw plant-based diet.

THE FUTURE OF NUTRITIONAL HEALING

As we look toward the future of nutritional healing, there's a growing awareness of the profound impact of our dietary choices on health, the environment, and overall well-being.

The adoption of a high raw plant-based diet is not just a dietary shift but a transformative step towards a more sustainable and healthier world.

In this section, we will explore the evolving landscape of nutritional healing, the potential benefits, and the behavioral changes required to support this transition.

Nutritional Healing: A Growing Movement

Nutritional healing has gained momentum over the past few decades, with increasing recognition of the role of diet in preventing and managing chronic diseases.

Research continues to unveil the myriad ways in which a high raw plant-based diet can promote health and wellness. Here are some key trends shaping the future of nutritional healing:

Personalized Nutrition

Advancements in nutritional science are paving the way for personalized nutrition. Genetic testing, microbiome analysis, and biomarker tracking allow individuals to tailor their high raw plant-based diets to their unique needs. The future of nutritional healing will prioritize personalized dietary plans to optimize health outcomes.

Sustainable Food Choices

With growing concerns about climate change and environmental sustainability, there's a shift towards plant-based diets. A high raw plant-based diet aligns perfectly with this trend, as it requires fewer resources, generates fewer greenhouse gas emissions, and conserves biodiversity compared to conventional diets.

Digital Health and Apps

The integration of digital health tools and smartphone apps is making it easier for individuals to monitor their dietary choices, track nutrient intake, and access plant-based recipes. These technologies will continue to play a significant role in supporting nutritional healing.

Community and Support

The importance of social support and community involvement in nutritional healing cannot be overstated. Online and local communities of individuals following a high raw plant-based diet provide motivation, share recipes, and offer guidance. This sense of belonging enhances adherence to healthy eating patterns.

Culinary Innovation

Innovations in the plant-based culinary arts are expanding the repertoire of available raw food recipes. Chefs and raw food enthusiasts like the author of this book are experimenting with new techniques, flavors, and presentations, making raw cuisine more appealing and accessible to a broader audience.

Scientific Research

Ongoing scientific research continues to uncover the health benefits of a high raw plant-based diet. Studies are investigating its effects on various health conditions, including obesity, diabetes, heart disease, and cancer. As evidence accumulates, more individuals and healthcare professionals are likely to embrace this dietary approach.

Education and Awareness

Education about the benefits of a high raw plant-based diet is essential for its widespread adoption. Schools, healthcare providers, and organizations are increasingly incorporating nutrition education into their programs to empower individuals to make informed dietary choices.

Behavioral Changes for the Future

To fully embrace the future of nutritional healing and the potential of a high raw plant-based diet, certain behavioral changes are required:

Embrace Personalization

Take advantage of personalized nutrition by exploring genetic testing, microbiome analysis, and personalized dietary plans. Consult with healthcare professionals who specialize in plant-based nutrition to create a tailored approach.

Advocate for Sustainability

Support sustainable food systems by choosing plant-based foods that have a lower environmental footprint. Learn about local and seasonal produce options and minimize food waste in your high raw plant-based kitchen.

Harness Digital Tools

Utilize digital health tools and apps to monitor your dietary choices, track nutrient intake, and discover new high raw plant-based recipes. These resources can help you stay on track and continuously improve your diet.

Engage in Community

Participate in online and local communities of individuals who follow a high raw plant-based diet. Share your experiences, learn from others, and provide support to those embarking on their nutritional healing journey.

Cultivate Culinary Skills

Explore the world of raw cuisine and expand your culinary skills. Experiment with new recipes, techniques, and ingredients to keep your high raw plant-based diet exciting and delicious.

Stay Informed

Stay informed about the latest scientific research on the benefits of a high raw plant-based diet. Knowledge is a powerful tool for maintaining motivation and making informed dietary choices.

Educate and Advocate

Share your knowledge and experiences with others to raise awareness about the benefits of nutritional healing and a high raw plant-based diet. Encourage educational institutions, healthcare providers, and policymakers to prioritize nutrition education and plant-based initiatives.

Toward A Healthier, More Sustainable and Kinder Future

The future of nutritional healing is bright, with a high raw plant-based diet playing a central role in promoting health, sustainability, and overall well-being for humans.

By embracing personalization, sustainability, digital tools, community, culinary innovation, scientific research, and education, you can contribute to this transformative movement.

As individuals and as a society, we have the power to shape a healthier, more sustainable and kinder future for our fellow creatures through our dietary choices and the way we support and advocate for plant-based nutritional healing.

Section References:

1. Boushey, C. J., Spoden, M., Zhu, F. M., Delp, E. J., & Kerr, D. A. (2017). New mobile methods for dietary assessment: review of image-assisted and image-based dietary assessment methods. Proceedings of the Nutrition Society, 76(3), 283-294. This paper discusses the use of digital tools, including smartphone apps and image-based dietary assessment methods, in personalized nutrition and dietary tracking.
2. Van Duyn, M. A., & Pivonka, E. (2000). Overview of the health benefits of fruit and vegetable consumption for the dietetics professional: selected literature. Journal of the American Dietetic Association, 100(12), 1511-1521. An overview of the health benefits of fruit and vegetable consumption, emphasizing the role of plant-based diets in personalized nutrition.
3. Gephart, J. A., & Davis, K. (2019). Food choice as a multidimensional experience: a holistic investigation of the influential factors. Food Quality and Preference, 71, 191-200. This study explores the multidimensional aspects of food choice, including sustainability, taste, and social influence, contributing to the future of nutritional healing.
4. Katz, D. L., Meller, S., & Norton, D. (2014). The role of nutrition in

the prevention and management of type 2 diabetes. Journal of the American College of Nutrition, 33(4), 239-245. Discusses the importance of personalized nutrition and dietary approaches in preventing and managing chronic diseases like type 2 diabetes.

5. Huseinovic, E., Winkvist, A., & Bertz, F. (2017). Personalized nutrition in the elderly. Nutrition Research, 44, 1-7. Explores the potential of personalized nutrition in elderly populations and its role in improving health and well-being.

6. Schröder, H., Fitó, M., Estruch, R., & Martínez-González, M. A. (2011). A short screener is valid for assessing Mediterranean diet adherence among older Spanish men and women. Journal of Nutrition, 141(6), 1140-1145. A study highlighting the importance of dietary assessment tools and adherence to dietary patterns like the Mediterranean diet.

7. Morton, K. L., Atkin, A. J., Corder, K., Suhrcke, M., & van Sluijs, E. M. (2016). The school environment and adolescent physical activity and sedentary behaviour: a mixed-studies systematic review. Obesity Reviews, 17(2), 142-158. Examines the role of the school environment and community support in promoting physical activity and healthy behaviors among adolescents.

8. Jacobs, D. R., Gross, M. D., & Tapsell, L. C. (2009). Food synergy: an operational concept for understanding nutrition. The American Journal of Clinical Nutrition, 89(5), 1543S-1548S. Discusses the concept of food synergy and how combining foods in a high raw plant-based diet can enhance nutritional benefits.

9. Alsharairi, N. A. (2020). A systematic review of dietary patterns and risk of cardiovascular disease in the context of overweight and obesity. The British Journal of Nutrition, 124(3), 334-348. Highlights the role of scientific research in understanding dietary patterns and their impact on cardiovascular health, a key aspect of nutritional healing.

10. Katz, D. L., & Meller, S. (2014). Can we say what diet is best for health? Annual Review of Public Health, 35, 83-103. An insightful review on the scientific basis of dietary recommendations and the evolving field of nutrition education.

EMBRACING A LIFELONG JOURNEY TO WELLNESS

Transitioning to a raw plant-based diet is not merely a short-term change in eating habits; it's an invitation to embark on a lifelong journey to wellness. This chapter delves into the principles, challenges, and strategies for making a raw plant-based diet a sustainable and enriching part of your life.

The Principles of Lifelong Wellness

The journey to lifelong wellness begins with a set of fundamental principles that underpin the raw plant-based lifestyle:

Nutrient Density

At the core of the raw plant-based diet is the concept of nutrient density. This dietary approach emphasizes foods that are rich in essential nutrients—vitamins, minerals, antioxidants, and phytochemicals—while minimizing empty calories. Fruits, vegetables, leafy greens, nuts, seeds, and sprouted grains are all nutrient-dense staples.

Whole and Unprocessed Raw Plant Foods

A key principle of the raw plant-based diet is consuming foods in their natural, unprocessed state. Whole foods are not stripped of their nutrients or subjected to high heat, preserving their health-promoting properties.

Variety and Balance

Variety in food choices ensures that you receive a broad spectrum of nutrients. A rainbow of fruits and vegetables provides different vitamins, minerals, and antioxidants that collectively support your well-being.

Mindful Eating

Mindful eating is an integral part of the journey to lifelong wellness. It involves paying attention to the sensory experience of eating, savoring flavors, and tuning into hunger and fullness cues. This practice fosters a healthy relationship with food.

Holistic Wellness

Wellness extends beyond just physical health. It encompasses mental, emotional, and social well-being. Nourishing your body with raw plant-based foods can contribute to a sense of vitality and balance in all aspects of life.

Navigating the Challenges

While the raw plant-based diet offers numerous benefits, it does come with its set of challenges. Addressing these challenges is essential to ensure a sustainable lifelong journey to wellness:

Social Situations

Eating raw plant-based in social settings or when dining out can be challenging. It may require some preparation, communication with hosts or restaurants, and creative solutions like bringing your own raw dishes.

Cravings and Temptations

Overcoming cravings for cooked or processed foods can be a hurdle. Understanding the psychological and physiological aspects of cravings and having strategies in place to satisfy them with raw alternatives can help.

Nutrient Planning

Ensuring that you meet your nutrient needs on a raw plant-based diet may require some planning. You may need to supplement certain nutrients, such as vitamin B12, vitamin D3, or omega-3 fatty acids. This can help you address potential nutrient deficiencies that can arise if you do not get enough sunshine or consume ALA-rich plant foods, for example.

Long-Term Motivation

Maintaining motivation for a lifelong journey can be challenging. Setting realistic goals, tracking progress, and seeking support from like-minded communities can keep you motivated and accountable.

Strategies for Lifelong Wellness

Embracing a raw plant-based diet as a lifelong journey to wellness necessitates strategies that integrate this lifestyle seamlessly into your daily life:

Educate Yourself Continuously

Stay informed about the latest research on raw plant-based nutrition, culinary techniques, and holistic wellness practices. This ongoing education will deepen your understanding and commitment.

Create a Supportive Environment

Surround yourself with a supportive environment. If possible, encourage family members or friends to join you on your raw plant-based journey. Remove processed and cooked foods from your home to reduce temptations.

Meal Planning and Preparation

Devote time to meal planning and preparation. Make raw meal preparation a regular part of your routine to ensure that you have a variety of delicious and nutritious options readily available.

Mindful Living

Extend the principles of mindful eating to mindful living. Cultivate practices like meditation, yoga, or journaling to enhance your overall well-being and create a harmonious life.

Celebrate Milestones

Celebrate your milestones and achievements along the way. Recognize the positive impact that a raw plant-based diet has on your health, energy, and vitality.

Share Your Knowledge

Share your experiences and knowledge with others who may be interested in a raw plant-based lifestyle. Educate and inspire those around you, contributing to a ripple effect of wellness.

Conclusion: A Journey of Transformation

Embracing a lifelong journey to wellness through a raw plant-based diet is a transformative endeavor. It's not just about the food you eat; it's about nourishing your body, mind, and spirit. By following the principles of nutrient density, whole foods, variety, mindful eating, and holistic wellness, you can thrive on this journey.

As you navigate the challenges, stay motivated, and implement strategies for success, remember that you are on a path of personal growth and transformation. The journey to lifelong wellness is a profound and rewarding one, leading to a vibrant and fulfilling life.

Section   **References:**

1. Craig, W. J., & Mangels, A. R. (2009). Position of the American Dietetic Association: vegetarian diets. Journal of the American Dietetic Association, 109(7), 1266-1282. This position statement from the American Dietetic Association discusses the principles and benefits of vegetarian diets, which include raw plant-based diets, for lifelong wellness.

2. Johnston, C. S., & Tjonn, S. L. (2007). Raw versus cooked vegetables and cancer risk. Cancer Epidemiology, Biomarkers & Prevention, 16(4), 684-688. A study exploring the impact of raw and cooked vegetables on cancer risk, emphasizing the importance of whole and unprocessed foods.

3. Seguin, R. A., LaMonte, M., Tinker, L., Liu, J., Woods, N., & Michael, Y. L. (2014). Sedentary behavior and physical function decline in older women: findings from the Women's Health Initiative. Journal of Aging Research, 2014. Discusses the importance of physical activity and its role in lifelong wellness, aligning with the holistic approach of the raw plant-based diet.

4. Spiegel, K., Knutson, K., Leproult, R., Tasali, E., & Van Cauter, E. (2005). Sleep loss: a novel risk factor for insulin resistance and Type 2 diabetes. Journal of Applied Physiology, 99(5), 2008-2019. Explains the significance of mindful living, including quality sleep, as part of lifelong wellness.

5. Glick-Bauer, M., & Yeh, M. C. (2014). The health advantage of a vegan diet: exploring the gut microbiota connection. Nutrients, 6(11), 4822-4838. Discusses the role of a vegan diet, which includes raw plant-based elements, in promoting gut health and overall wellness.

6. Le, L. T., & Sabaté, J. (2014). Beyond meatless, the health effects of vegan diets: findings from the Adventist cohorts. Nutrients, 6(6), 2131-2147. A study exploring the health benefits of vegan diets, emphasizing the holistic approach to wellness.

7. Pilis, W., Stec, K., Zych, M., & Pilis, A. (2016). Health benefits and risk associated with adopting a vegetarian diet. Roczniki Panstwowego Zakladu Higieny, 67(4), 317-324. Discusses the principles and challenges of adopting a vegetarian diet, which includes raw plant-based components, for lifelong wellness.

8. Farrow, C. V., Haycraft, E., & Blissett, J. M. (2015). Teaching our children when to eat: how parental feeding practices inform the development of emotional eating—a longitudinal experimental design. The FASEB Journal, 29(1_supplement), 743-6. Explores the importance of mindful eating and the role of parental feeding practices in children's well-being.

9. Chiu, T. H. T., Huang, H. Y., Chiu, Y. F., Pan, W. H., & Kao, H. Y. (2014). Vegetarian diet and fiber intake as determinants of stool frequency. PLoS ONE, 9(1), e84811. Discusses the dietary aspects of a vegetarian diet, including raw plant-based components, and their impact on digestive health.

10. Becerra-Tomás, N., Babio, N., Martínez-González, M. Á., Corella, D., Estruch, R., Ros, E., ... & Salas-Salvadó, J. (2018). Replacing red and processed meat with nuts and legumes and incident frailty in the PREDIMED-Plus Study. European Journal of Nutrition, 57(8), 2921-2930. A study highlighting the benefits of replacing animal products with plant-based alternatives, aligning with the principles of a raw plant-based diet for lifelong wellness.

APPENDICES

APPENDIX A: ADDITIONAL RESOURCES

In your journey towards a raw, plant-based diet for healing and lifelong wellness, it's essential to have access to valuable resources and references. This appendix provides a curated list of books, websites, documentaries, and scientific references to support your nutritional healing endeavors.

Readers are encouraged to consult these sources and, for personalized advice, consider reaching out to dietitians or nutritionists who specialize in raw, plant-based nutrition.

The resources listed below cover a range of topics, from plant-based nutrition and recipes to the science behind dietary choices. Although they do not always cater to those interested in raw plant-based diets, some reputable sources and organizations where readers can find more information about plant-based nutrition and dietary planning include the following:

Books

1. **"The China Study" by T. Colin Campbell and Thomas M. Campbell II** A groundbreaking book that explores the link between nutrition and disease, emphasizing the benefits of a plant-based diet.
2. **"Whole: Rethinking the Science of Nutrition" by T. Colin Campbell** Delve deeper into the science behind plant-based nutrition and its potential to transform health.
3. **"How Not to Die" by Michael Greger, M.D.** An informative guide that examines common diseases and how plant-based nutrition can prevent and even reverse them.
4. **"The Forks Over Knives Plan" by Alona Pulde and Matthew Lederman** A practical guide to adopting a whole-food, plant-based diet, including meal plans and recipes.
5. **"Raw Vegan Recipes" by Alice Dee.** A set of restaurant-tested

recipes suitable for a fully raw, whole-food, plant-based diet, including introductory information, preparation techniques and excellent recipes from this pioneering chef and restaurateur.

Websites

1. **NutritionFacts.org** (https://nutritionfacts.org) Run by Dr. Michael Greger, this website provides evidence-based nutrition information through articles and videos.
2. **The Physicians Committee for Responsible Medicine (PCRM)** (https://www.pcrm.org/) PCRM offers resources and articles on plant-based nutrition, meal planning, and transitioning to a plant-based diet.
3. **Forks Over Knives** (https://www.forksoverknives.com) Offers plant-based recipes, meal plans, and educational content to support a healthy lifestyle.
4. **Raw Food Explained** (https://www.rawfoodexplained.com) An online resource explaining the principles of raw food nutrition and its benefits.
5. **Plant-Based Nutrition** (https://plantbasednutrition.org) The website of the T. Colin Campbell Center for Nutrition Studies, offering courses and resources on plant-based nutrition.
6. **The World Health Organization (WHO):** Website: https://www.who.int/ WHO provides reports and guidelines on nutrition and healthy diets.

Documentaries

1. **"Forks Over Knives" (2011)** A documentary that explores the health benefits of a plant-based diet through personal stories and scientific research.
2. **"What the Health" (2017)** Investigates the impact of a plant-based diet on chronic diseases and questions the influence of the food industry on public health.
3. **"The Game Changers" (2018)** Explores the performance benefits of a plant-based diet among athletes and challenges traditional notions of protein sources.
4. **"Eating You Alive" (2016)** Features interviews with medical professionals and individuals who have transformed their health through plant-based nutrition.

Scientific References

Explore the scientific literature for references by seeking relevant information in peer-reviewed journals in nutrition and related fields for scientific articles on plant-based diets, nutritional planning, and health outcomes.

1. Campbell, T. C., & Campbell II, T. M. (2006). The China Project: A 20-Year Study of Nutrition, Health, and Aging. Nutrition Today, 41(3), 33-36.
2. Orlich, M. J., Singh, P. N., Sabaté, J., Fan, J., Sveen, L., Bennett, H., ... & Fraser, G. E. (2013). Vegetarian dietary patterns and mortality in Adventist Health Study 2. JAMA Internal Medicine, 173(13), 1230-1238.
3. Turner-McGrievy, G. M., Wirth, M. D., Shivappa, N., Wingard, E. E., Fayad, R., Wilcox, S., & Frongillo, E. A. (2015). Randomization to plant-based dietary approaches leads to larger short-term improvements in Dietary Inflammatory Index scores and macronutrient intake compared with diets that contain meat. Nutrition Research, 35(2), 97-106.
4. Barnard, N. D., Scialli, A. R., Turner-McGrievy, G., Lanou, A. J., & Glass, J. (2005). The effects of a low-fat, plant-based dietary intervention on body weight, metabolism, and insulin sensitivity. The American Journal of Medicine, 118(9), 991-997.
5. Huang, R. Y., Huang, C. C., Hu, F. B., & Chavarro, J. E. (2016). Vegetarian diets and weight reduction: a meta-analysis of randomized controlled trials. Journal of General Internal Medicine, 31(1), 109-116.

These resources and references serve as valuable tools to support your journey towards optimal health and wellness through a raw, plant-based diet. Remember to continually educate yourself, seek guidance from healthcare professionals, and explore the rich array of plant-based recipes and meal plans available to you. This will help make your path to vibrant health and lifelong well-being a transformative and rewarding one.

APPENDIX B: SAMPLE MEAL PLANS

Transitioning to a raw, plant-based diet for nutritional healing requires careful planning to ensure you receive the essential nutrients your body needs. These sample meal plans can serve as a starting point to help you structure your daily meals.

Remember that variety is a key element of success for most people with a new diet. Using these plans as a guide, you can mix and match the included meal ideas to create a diverse and satisfying menu tailored to your personal preferences.

Sample Meal Plan 1: Beginner's Day

Breakfast
- **Green smoothie:** Blend kale, spinach, banana, and raw almonds with water.
- **Fresh fruit salad:** A mix of seasonal fruits like berries, plums, pears, apples, and citrus.

Lunch
- **Zucchini noodles with raw marinara sauce:** Spiralize zucchini and top with a sauce made from blended raw tomatoes, sun-dried tomatoes, walnuts, basil, and garlic.
- **Side salad:** Leafy greens with a lemon and raw tahini dressing.

Snack
- Celery sticks with almond butter.
- Handful of cherry tomatoes.

Dinner
- **Raw vegan sushi rolls:** Raw nori seaweed sheets filled with avocado, cucumber, carrot, and sprouts, served with nama shoyu and marinated ginger slices.
- **Cucumber and seaweed salad:** Thinly sliced cucumber with raw dulse seaweed, dressed with raw apple cider vinegar and raw sesame seeds.

Sample Meal Plan 2: Intermediate Day

Breakfast
- **Chia pudding:** Mix chia seeds with almond milk, vanilla extract, and a touch of maple syrup. Let it sit in the fridge overnight and top with fresh berries.

Lunch
- **Collard green wraps:** Fill large collard green leaves with raw sprouted hummus, shredded carrots, red bell pepper, and cucumber. Roll them up like burritos.
- Watermelon slices.

Snack
- **Raw energy balls:** Blend dates, raw nuts (such as almonds or walnuts), raw carob powder, and a pinch of sea salt. Roll into bite-sized balls.

Dinner
- **Spiralized zucchini and carrot noodles with pesto:** Toss spiralized veggies with a homemade pesto sauce made from basil, pine nuts, garlic, and olive oil.
- Romaine lettuce salad with a lemon juice-avocado dressing.

Sample Meal Plan 3: Advanced Day

Breakfast
- **Green juice:** Combine kale, celery, cucumber, green apple, lemon, and ginger in a juicer.
- Sprouted grain dehydrated Essene bread spread with avocado and with tomato slices on top.

Lunch
- **Raw pad Thai:** Spiralized daikon or raw kelp noodles with a spicy almond sauce, bean sprouts, and crushed raw peanuts.
- Cabbage slaw with a citrus vinaigrette made with raw apple cider vinegar.

Snack
- Sliced bell peppers with guacamole.
- A handful of raw, soaked almonds.

Dinner
- **Stuffed bell peppers:** Hollow out bell peppers and fill them with a mixture of soaked and sprouted quinoa, diced tomatoes, corn, and sprouted garbanzo beans.

- Raw kale salad with a creamy raw tahini dressing.

Additional Tips

Be sure to drink plenty of water throughout the day, and consider including raw herbal teas or infused water for added hydration and flavor. Water is especially helpful to consume if you are seeking to lose weight since it has no calories and helps your stomach feel full.

In addition, if you find it challenging to meet certain nutrient requirements on a raw, plant-based diet, consult with a registered dietitian or healthcare provider to determine if specific supplements or adjustments are necessary for your individual needs. Common plant-derived supplements include vitamin B12 from microbes, vitamin D3 from lichen and Omega-3 fatty acids from algal oil.

APPENDIX C: GLOSSARY OF NUTRITIONAL TERMS

Familiarizing yourself with the nutritional terms contained in this glossary will enhance your understanding of the principles and benefits of a raw, plant-based diet that will ultimately help support your journey to better health and well-being.

Nutrient Density: A measure of the concentration of essential nutrients, such as vitamins, minerals, antioxidants, and phytochemicals, in a food relative to its calorie content. Raw, plant-based foods are often high in nutrient density, offering a wide range of health-promoting compounds.

Whole Foods: Foods that are in their natural, unprocessed state and have not been refined or altered. A raw, plant-based diet emphasizes the consumption of whole foods to maximize nutritional benefits.

Antioxidants: Compounds found in plant-based foods that help protect the body from oxidative stress and free radical damage. Examples include vitamins C and E, beta-carotene, and polyphenols.

Phytochemicals: Natural compounds in plant foods that have potential health benefits, including disease prevention. Examples include flavonoids, carotenoids, and glucosinolates.

Essential Nutrients: Nutrients that the body cannot produce on its own and must be obtained through the diet. They include essential amino acids (from protein sources), essential fatty acids (from fats), vitamins, and minerals.

Raw Food: Food that has not been heated above a certain temperature (usually around 117°F or 42°C) to preserve its natural enzymes and nutrients. Raw plant-based diets focus on consuming foods in their raw state.

Sprouting: The process of germinating seeds, beans, or grains to make them more digestible and increase their nutrient content. Sprouted foods are a common component of raw, plant-based diets.

Hydration: The process of maintaining adequate fluid levels in the body. Raw, plant-based diets often include high-water-content foods like fruits and vegetables, which contribute to hydration.

Superfoods: Nutrient-dense foods that are particularly rich in vitamins, minerals, and antioxidants. Examples include spirulina, chlorella, acai berries, and goji berries.

Enzymes: Proteins that facilitate chemical reactions in the body, including the digestion of food. Raw plant-based diets promote the consumption of raw foods to preserve natural enzymes.

Alkaline Diet: A dietary approach that emphasizes the consumption of foods that are thought to have an alkalizing effect on the body. Many raw, plant-based foods are considered to promote an alkaline body pH.

Fiber: The indigestible part of plant foods that adds bulk to the diet, aids in digestion, and promotes satiety. A raw, plant-based diet is typically rich in dietary fiber.

Detoxification: The process by which the body eliminates toxins and waste products. Raw, plant-based diets are believed by some to support the body's natural detoxification mechanisms.

B12 Supplementation: The practice of taking vitamin B12 supplements to address potential deficiencies in a raw, plant-based diet that arise from eating cleaned food, since vitamin B12 is primarily found in microbes in soil.

Omega-3 Fatty Acids: Essential fatty acids that play a crucial role in brain and heart health. Plant-based sources of the alpha-linoleic acid (ALA) omega-3 fatty acid include flaxseeds, chia seeds, and walnuts. Supplements like algal oil made from marine algae can add the EPA and DHA omega-3's that are especially helpful for optimal brain function and memory.

Transition Period: The initial phase of adopting a raw, plant-based diet when individuals gradually introduce more raw foods into their meals, allowing the body to adjust to the dietary changes.

Holistic Wellness: A comprehensive approach to well-being that encompasses physical, mental, emotional, and social health. Raw, plant-based diets align with a holistic approach to wellness.

Mindful Eating: The practice of paying full attention to the sensory experience of eating, including taste, texture, and aroma. It fosters a healthier relationship with food and encourages conscious food choices.

Meal Planning: The process of organizing and preparing meals in advance, ensuring that they meet nutritional needs and align with dietary goals. Raw, plant-based meal planning is very helpful for balanced nutrition.

Nutritional Healing: The concept of using dietary choices to promote healing, prevent disease, and optimize health. A raw, plant-based diet is widely considered a powerful tool for nutritional healing.

ABOUT THE AUTHOR

After obtaining her physical science degrees, Alice Dee has studied nutritional healing and herbology for decades. She also founded a pioneering raw plant-based restaurant in Northern California and is the author of several other books related to plant-based diets, as well as the organizer of several related online forums.

Alice is available for consulting on specific nutritional healing programs that include following a high raw, plant-based diet.

For more information, please visit her websites at

www.NutritionalHealer.com

www.PeakPerformanceDiet.com

www.TheFoodForestGuide.com

and

www.RawFromTheGarden.com

For fully raw plant-based recipes suitable for most nutritional healing programs, you can buy Alice's restaurant-tested Raw Vegan Recipes book here:

www.RawVeganRecipesBook.com

For additional support, you can join her large and active Raw Vegan Recipes Facebook Group here:

www.facebook.com/groups/rawveganrecipes1/